Healing Cancer with the Nervous System

A New Concept to Understand Cancer

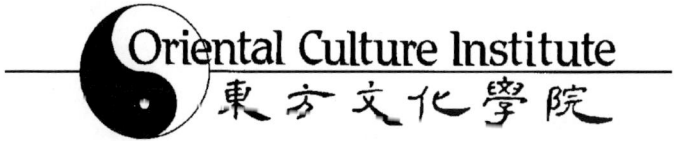

Tom Tam

Copyright © 2012 by Oriental Culture Institute

Published by Oriental Culture Institute

Illustrations by Michael Malbrough

Edited by Kathryn Marion

Printing by Expert Self Publishing

All rights reserved. No part of this publication may be reproduced, stored in a retrieval system or transmitted, in any form, or by any means, electronic, mechanical, recorded, photocopied, or otherwise, without the prior permission of the copyright owner, except by a reviewer who may quote brief passages in a review.

Printed in the United States of America

ISBN 978-0-9831023-0-4

LIMITS OF LIABILITY
DISCLAIMER OF WARRANTY

While all attempts have been made to verify the information provided in this publication, neither the authors nor the publisher assume any responsibility for errors, inaccuracies, or omissions. Any slights of people, groups or organizations are unintentional. This publication is not intended for use as a source of medical, legal, or professional information and should not be used as such. Rather, appropriate professionals should be consulted. All users of this information must be sure all appropriate Federal, State, and local laws and regulations are followed. The authors and publisher assume no responsibility or liability whatsoever on behalf of any purchaser, reader, or user of these materials. They disclaim any warranties (expressed or implied), merchantability, or fitness for any loss or other damages, including but not limited to special, incidental, consequential, or other damages.

Acknowledgements

Writing is not an easy job for me, especially since I did not finish junior high school in China and had only one year of English education in America. I consider myself fortunate to have had many students, patients, doctors, and even children help me with my writing. I am very appreciative of their help with my job of healing the world.

I sincerely thank all those who have helped me. Special thanks go to Dr. Jack Weltner M.D., Laura De Gregorio, Roni Bethell, Angie Lawless, Aimée W. Poirier Lic.Ac., Anita Galletti Lic.Ac., Tom Lee, Kathleen Kearney, Eleanor Marks Ph.D., and Yvonne Tam for their help with compiling this book.

Contents

Acknowledgements 3

Contents i

Foreword 1

To Understand Cancer, We Must Understand the Body 9

    A Forgotten Nervous System 13

    The Autonomic Nervous System 21

    The Nervous System's Function 23

    The Brain's Role 24

    Human Cells as Miniature Batteries 25

    Biochemistry vs. Bioelectricity 27

    Applying Ohm's Law to Human Bioelectricity 28

    Beyond Basic Anatomy: The Dantian and Shu Points 29

    Meridians are the Highway for *Chi* 32

San Jiao 37

Where and How Did the Meridian System Originate?
.... 44

Different Viewpoints on Meridians and the Nervous System 54

Free Radicals and the Kidney Meridian 59

  Free Radicals 61

  Free Radicals and Tong Ren Healing 77

  Telomere and Enzyme 82

Neocortex and Gallbladder Meridian 95

  So What is the Neocortex? 98

Discovering the Cause of Cancer 113

  Warburg's Findings Gain Attention 117

  Trying to Unlock the Cause of Cancer 119

  Does DNA Play a Role? 120

  Can the Somatic Nervous System Cause Cancer?
  123

  Can the Vascular System Cause Cancer? 124

  What about Mineral Supplements? 127

  Arteries of Systemic Circulation 128

How Does Diet Fit In? 130

The Future of Cancer Research 131

Preventing Cancer 133

    Do Supplements Have a Place in Cancer Prevention? 133

    A Cancer-Preventing Diet 134

    Exercise as a Cancer Preventative 135

    Preventing Colorectal Cancer 136

Healing Cancer 141

    Misguided Treatments for Healing Cancer 141

    Drug Companies and Doctors Focus on the Wrong Areas 143

    The Diaphragm is Unique 145

    Focus on the Diaphragm for Healing 146

    Bioelectricity's Role in Healing Cancer 148

    The Spinal Column's Role in Healing Cancer 151

    The Role of Chi in Healing Cancer 154

    Locating Blockage Points for Use in Healing 154

    Using These Points to Heal Cancer 162

Diet and Cancer Healing 163

Healing Genetic Cancers 167

Can Patients Fight Against Cancer? 169

Are the "Big Three" Effective in Healing Cancer?. 171

Beyond the "Big Three" 175

The Tom Tam Healing System 177

Tong Ren Healing 180

Finding Blockages is Key 183

Healing Specific Cancers 185

Pancreatic Cancer 185

Breast Cancer 196

Colon Cancer 207

Lung Cancer 217

Leukemia 231

Tong Ren for Cancer Simple Point Chart 240

Using this Theory for Healing Cancer 244

Poll of Tong Ren Healing for Cancer 248

Afterword 263

Foreword

Ten years ago, I wrote my first book about healing cancer, *Tong Ren for Cancer*. In that book, the healing theory for cancer focused on bioelectricity and the autonomic nervous system. My students and I used this theory to successfully heal many cancer patients. Now it is time to update it with exciting new data.

Today, I have learned about another factor that can cause cancer: oxygen deficiency. This theory is not from my own studies, but from 1931 Nobel Prize winner, Dr. Otto H. Warburg. Many experts have their own opinions about Warburg's theory and use it for different healing purposes. I, too, have my own understanding and use his theory in my practice for healing cancer.

In the last 50 years, the research on healing cancer has focused on chemical and/or radiological approaches. Who knows how much money has been invested and how many people have died from cancer and cancer "treatments"? Yet, few will change their mind about these approaches.

New chemotherapy drugs continue to be developed. Each month we hear about new chemical drugs claiming to "heal" cancer. Unfortunately, too many people believe that these products can, in fact, heal their cancer.

Countless stage-4 cancer patients who have given up hope after using the "Big Three" for treatment believe that the only possible next step is to participate in a clinical trial. But how much do these patients really know about those trials? Do they ask questions, or do they passively assume that it is the logical, and only, next step? In their minds, there seems to be no choice—participating in a clinical trial sounds better than being told that they are waiting to die.

These trials are testing chemical treatments—but are any non-chemical trials available? This may sound like a joke or a daydream. Who has the ability, funding, and willingness to support such a trial? Will pharmaceutical companies or insurance companies support trials using non-chemical-based healing methods?

According to the Hippocratic Oath, "without doing harm," a 'clinical trial' *should* mean the open, scientific search for *any* method that can promote the healing of cancer. Logically, when drugs cannot help, then a *non*-chemical solution should be explored. Many thousands of chemotherapy formulations have produced terrible side-effects, or even caused the *spread* of cancer by knocking down the patients' immune systems, yet the pharmaceutical pipeline of research continues. The medical community is very stubborn—when one drug does not help, they unquestioningly continue their search by trying others.

How many patients benefit from these new drugs? How many suffer harm from them? How many of them can survive new medication protocols, and how long can they survive? There are so many questions about clinical trials, yet, who actually questions whether they can heal cancer or help patients who are suffering?

While most scientists are in favor of studying the effectiveness of chemicals for healing cancer, another practical theory is emerging. Tong Ren healing believes that cancer is caused by bioelectrical dysfunction; in other words, *the nervous system causes cancer.*

In human physiology, there are two physical functions: biochemical and bioelectrical. If we cannot understand the cause of cancer from the biochemistry side, we should investigate how bioelectricity might contribute. This is common sense.

Otto Warburg believed that the primary cause of cancer is oxygen deficiency. Tong Ren's healing philosophy believes this is due to a dysfunction of the phrenic nerve and autonomic nervous system.

To heal cancer, we must use knowledge from traditional Western science to understand the body and the disease. However, the West lacks knowledge of energy points and blockages as they relate to the nervous system. Combining these two healing systems, however, we can finally resolve this problem and truly heal cancer.

Historically, this is the first time that a new concept—a new medical theory—has pointed to the nervous system as the cause of cancer. Of course, any new concept, especially as it gains visibility, will be attacked by critics. In the last few years, scientists and doctors who are self-proclaimed skeptics have attacked Tong Ren healing over the radio, over the Internet, or in their magazines.

True scientists or healers don't worry about this criticism. We, the Tong Ren practitioners, will never give up the practice because we have helped so many 'hopeless' and 'untreatable' patients return to their normal lives. Confidently, we can see the future: Tong Ren healing will be popular because it *works*.

Scientists should realize that there is not just one answer to any health problem. If you are a cancer expert, healer, or researcher, aren't you tired of a job that's wasting your time? Studying science should be a challenge, but it can also be enjoyable— enjoying a carefree, open mind continually searching widely and creatively for better results. If one path leads to a dead end, will you turn back to find a new one or keep moving on blindly in the same direction? If the blockage of bioelectricity reduces oxygen to the cells and in fact causes cancer, how can we prove it's true or false until we have the support to do longitudinal experimental studies?

Tong Ren practitioners are the first to study the nervous system in regards to the causation of cancer. People may laugh at this 'crazy' new concept of healing cancer, but it is a challenge that offers a new way of thinking to the medical field.

Tong Ren is increasing in popularity as more people accept this new science. Our doors are open to anyone interested in what we do or who are in need of our help. Science needs fearless observers, so, we do not fear our critics. We do not want to argue with the skeptics, and we should not label them as 'bad' people. In fact, we should be sympathetic towards them because I believe they have a problem called Neophobia (the fear of new things). Neophobics prefer repetition, routine, and predictability—and that is how the general medical field carries out its approach to studying cancer.

As Science has become more complex and health care more uncertain, this phobia has become epidemic. As Dr. Larry Dossey states in his book, *The Extra-Ordinary Healing Power of Ordinary Things*: "There is a strange coterie of humans who devote their lives to attacking what they consider the irrational beliefs of others, often with great fanfare. Although they refer to themselves as skeptics, this term is misleading and far too flattering. 'Skeptic' is from the Greek word *skeptikos*, meaning 'thoughtful, inquiring.' A genuine skeptic according to Webster's is 'a person who habitually doubts, questions, or suspends judgment upon matters generally accepted.' Skepticism is a valuable and an honored tradition within science and science cannot thrive without it. However, individuals who loath miracles and assault those who believe in them are untrue to authentic skepticism, because they do not suspend judgment; their minds are already made up."

Traditional approaches to health care are becoming more closely scrutinized as many patients look for complementary means of dealing with the source of their illness. Interestingly, research is showing that seventy percent of all illnesses have a psychological source, with stress being the leading factor.

Looking forward, Tong Ren will undoubtedly transform the medical mainstream due to its remarkable healing results and substantive scientific theories. There will be no more neophobia and no more Skeptics. We are all friends, and are healing the world together. Let this book open your eyes to this exciting new healing theory.

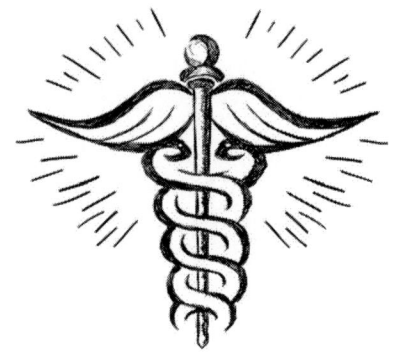

To Understand Cancer, We Must Understand the Body

There are many ways to heal cancer. From these, many healing theories and methods have been developed over the last 50 years. But can we really heal cancer or are these just theories to help calm down the psychological problem? When a person is diagnosed with any type of cancer, advice begins to pour in from others, non-stop, for emotional support. Yet, does all this advice really help or does it just come from sympathy, without being backed any experience or knowledge?

In fact, how many people, including the experts, have actually had their method heal cancer? Of course some people get healed from their cancer with an old or new method, but if we ask about the healing rate of that method, it is another story. To be healed is important, but a *repeatable* method to heal cancer is more important. Everyone knows that healing cancer must be proven in a scientific way, but the scientific knowledge we possess is limited. Everyone has their own view of looking at science even though we may have the same scientific knowledge.

Following scientific knowledge is the most important part of healing cancer. If we only have scientific knowledge, without common sense, then healing may not take effect with a good result. So far, medical studies have much knowledge about tumors and cells. This type of knowledge is only limited to the biochemical, based on commercial or political need, and does not form the whole picture. If one were to ask the medical expert about the bioelectricity of the cells, then that would be another story. There is no doubt that high-technology can make people easily understand more about the tumor and cell's structure and chemical form. How many experts have given their attention and interest to even *consider* the effects of bioelectricity?

Understanding the anatomy of the body is easy, but to *view* the anatomy of the body is *not* easy. For example, most experts see the body as a biochemical form but do not see the bioelectrical form. We cannot say that modern medicine doesn't have enough information about cancer cells and tumors. In fact, the only problem is that people favor the chemical form and structure of cancer. There are many PhDs and experts with biochemistry degrees, but how many of them are in the field of bioelectricity? If one day more experts learn to understand the science of bioelectricity, the curing of cancer will be an easy job.

Many societies and professional experts are focusing their attention on research to find a way to heal cancer, but, sadly, no one is going to realize what they are missing in their research. The most popular form of research is the study of *how to use chemicals* to destroy cancer cells and tumors. Other research is focused on how to destroy or kill cancer cells using any old or new technique. These theories are not only popular in the West, but are shared by many nations. For example, in China, when a person is diagnosed with cancer, the first step they take is to discover which herb or diet they should take (in other words, a chemical approach).

It is very often that we hear someone tell a story that energy healing techniques can heal some cancer cases. This energy healing may be from an energy healer, a religion healer, a Chi Gong master, or even a psychic healer. When people hear that energy healing can heal cancer, they often wonder: how can we really believe this? Not everyone needs to believe in it, but if we do the research, no one can deny the benefits of energy healing.

Western medicine does not have an energy healing system, but it would not be a difficult matter to develop one. Western medicine has enough knowledge about bioelectricity as well as thorough knowledge of the nervous system, which is the passageway of bioelectricity. I often wonder why Western medical society has shown no interest in energy healing and has paid such little attention (if any at all) to bioelectricity for healing cancer.

Each nation has their own beliefs and practices for energy healing, yet they are limited to their own healing rate results and have the problem of demonstrating repeatable results—mainly because the theories remain within the ancient philosophy. The ancient healing method can heal some of the sickness, but its healing rate and range still need to be proven, just as an old computer needs to be updated. To match ancient healing with modern medical philosophy is not an easy job. In China, the TCM experts try to put the meridian theory and the nervous system together, yet their work is far from done.

Every cell in the body functions as a battery which contains electrical power. When we view the battery, the most important function is the electrical current. In the study of cancer cells, the same should happen—we should focus on the bioelectricity, not on their chemical structure. In the body, each cell's function originates from an electrical impulse which is related to the nervous system. The body's function cannot be separated from the nervous system. If the nervous system passes a wrong impulse signal to a normal cell, it may cause cancer.

In the last twenty years of practice, I have focused all my attention on the nervous system for healing cancer. Of course, my study is a personal experience which has not yet been proven by formal medical research. I believe that I am the first one to believe that an out-of-balance nervous system can cause cancer. My study and theory about the cause of cancer does not follow the mainstream—I view cancer cells from another angle. I am not attempting to create a strange, new idea to get attention. I simply want to share my thoughts and ideas gained from my healing practice experience. Perhaps someday someone who has the ability and power to do formal research will be interested enough to study this further.

A Forgotten Nervous System

Modern medicine has a rich knowledge about anatomy and physiology. The nervous system consists of the brain, spinal cord, and a complex network of neurons. It monitors and coordinates internal organ function, responds to changes in the external environment, and is responsible for sending, receiving, and interpreting information from all parts of the body.

Healing Cancer with the Nervous System

The nervous system is the body's decision and communication center. Western medicine has divided the nervous system into two parts: the central nervous system and the peripheral nervous system—together they control every part of a human's daily life, from breathing and blinking to helping the brain memorize facts for a test. Nerves extend from the brain to the face, nose, ears, eyes, and spinal cord, and from the spinal cord to the rest of the body.

The **central nervous system** (CNS) consists of the brain and spinal cord. It is responsible for receiving and interpreting signals from the peripheral nervous system, and it sends out signals, either consciously or unconsciously, to the peripheral nervous system. The **peripheral nervous system** (PNS) includes two types of cells: sensory nerve cells and motor nerve cells. The *sensory nerve cells* carry information from internal organs and external stimuli to the central nervous system. *Motor nerve cells* carry information from the central nervous system to organs, muscles, and glands.

The peripheral nervous system is divided into the somatic nervous system and the autonomic nervous system. The **somatic nervous system** controls skeletal muscle as well as external sensory organs such as the skin. It is considered a voluntary system because its responses can be controlled by the conscious mind. The autonomic nervous system controls involuntary muscles, such as smooth and cardiac muscles. This system is also called the involuntary nervous system and is controlled by the unconscious mind.

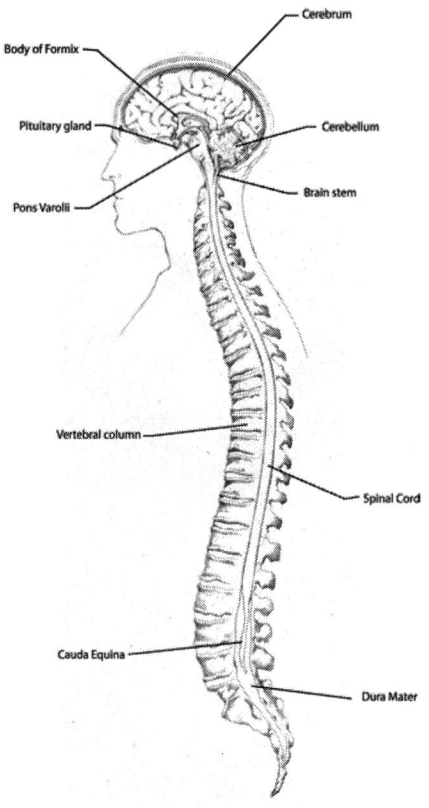

Central Nervous System

The **autonomic nervous system** has two divisions: parasympathetic nerves and sympathetic nerves. Organs which have a sympathetic nerve, must have a parasympathetic nerve as a complement, because these two nerves have an opposite effect.

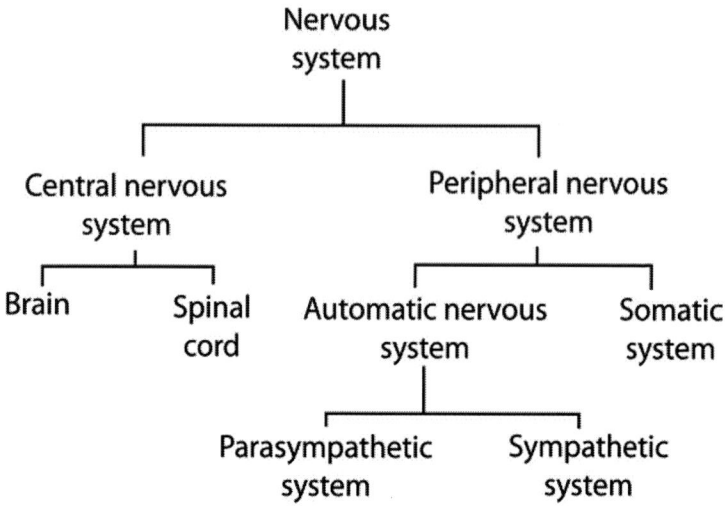

One nerve which belongs to the peripheral nervous system is of particular interest: the **phrenic nerve**. It contains motor, sensory, and sympathetic nerve fibers. These nerves provide the motor nerve conduction to the diaphragm as well as impulses to the central tendon. In the thorax, each phrenic nerve supplies the mediastinal pleura and pericardium with conductivity.

While the autonomic nerve is controlled by the unconscious mind and the motor nerve is controlled by the conscious mind, the phrenic nerve is controlled by both. It can also be controlled by the subconscious mind from life experience and breath training. It is difficult to see what system the phrenic nerve belongs to, but we believe it should be classified independently—in its own system, as a division of the peripheral nervous system.

From what we see in clinical practice, most doctors do not consider this nerve. Some surgeons may even damage this nerve unintentionally during surgery. Many medical experts have forgotten the phrenic nerve, because rarely can it be pinpointed as a factor in the diagnosis of any disease. It is used only for diagnostic check-ups or when addressing the cause of hiccups or injury.

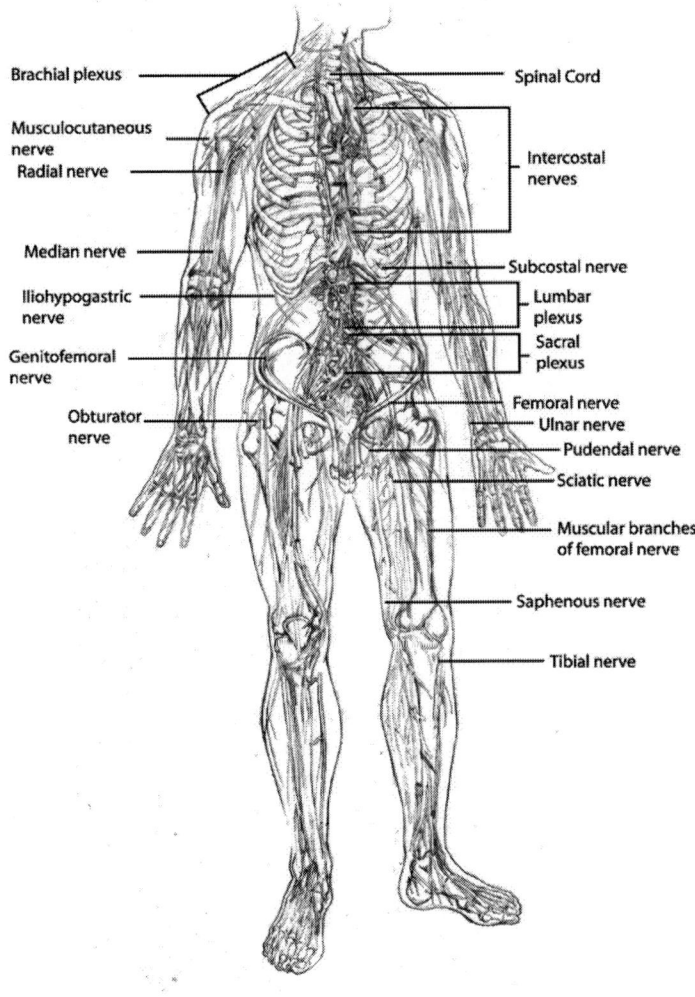

Another interesting nerve is the **accessory phrenic nerve**, which connects to the phrenic nerve. It joins the phrenic nerve either in the root of the neck or in the thorax, though most medical books have no information about it, and most doctors have never heard of it.

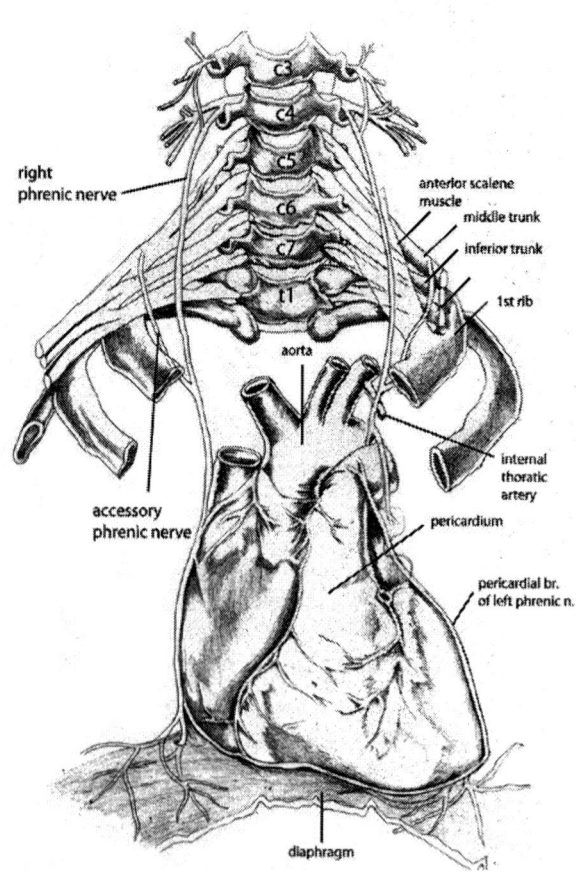

The phrenic nerve and the accessory phrenic nerve

We have discovered that only about half of all people have the accessory phrenic nerve, which is often located only on one side. Most people who have this nerve have only one, though some people may have three or even four branches of it. Why do some people have this nerve and some do not? Or why do some have one and some have many pathways of this nerve? To date, we do not have the answer to this question. We hope that someday scientists will conduct the research needed to answer this question so we can unlock the mysteries of these important nerves.

Through Western medical studies, we know that the life center is housed by the Medulla Oblongata, found in the brain stem. This life center includes the medullary rhythmicity center, the cardiac center, and vasomotor center, all of which function to control the level of oxygen within blood cells. The medulla passes impulses to the phrenic nerve which allows the diaphragm to function in a normal and healthy way. This means that the phrenic nerve is crucial to life force balance. If the phrenic nerve experiences a blockage or is out of balance, it may cause a problem of life force (i.e., disease).

In the study of TCM, the phrenic nerve is not mentioned. However, TCM practitioners know, in theory, the importance of the diaphragm. In the practice of Chi Gong, meditation, martial arts, Tai Chi, acupuncture, and even Chinese herbs and diet, much attention is paid to building up Chi in the Dantian, which is the diaphragm's function.

In Tong Ren healing, we often use the phrenic nerve to affect the metabolic system and breathing problems. We use it for healing cancer also, because cancer cells are formed by a metabolic system that is out of balance. Overweight people have a metabolism problem which may be caused by a lack of the oxygen needed to burn extra fat in the body. Because the phrenic nerve extends down to the liver, pericardium, bile duct, and lung area, we release the blockage of this nerve also when any of these organs is out of balance or dysfunctional.

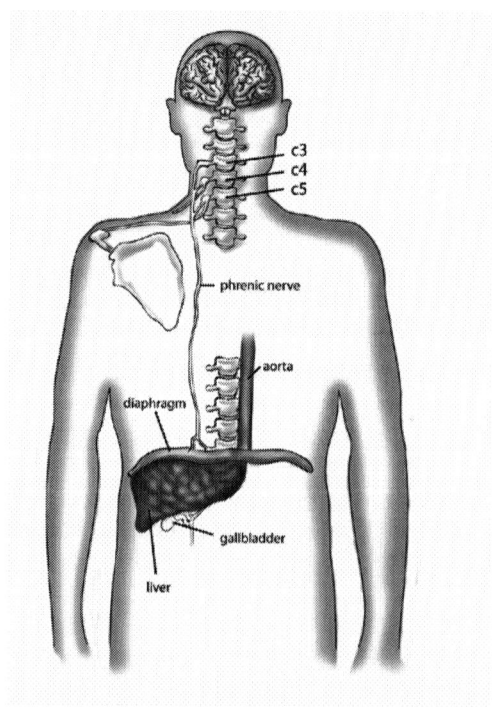

The Autonomic Nervous System

The **autonomic nervous system** (visceral nervous system) is formed by the parasympathetic nervous system and sympathetic nervous system. It is part of the peripheral nervous system that acts as a control system, functioning largely below the level of consciousness, and controls visceral, or organ, functions.

When the autonomic nerve has high resistance (called a blockage), it can cause a problem with impulses passing through it from the brain. The autonomic nervous system mainly affects heart rate, digestion, respiration rate, salivation, perspiration, diameter of the pupils, micturition (urination), and sexual arousal. Western medicine, however, does not acknowledge this function of the autonomic nervous system for any healing purpose.

If an organ has a blockage from its autonomic nerve, it means that organ lacks oxygen or there is a dysfunction with its oxygen. At times, understanding the result of the blockage can be difficult. A blockage does *not* necessarily mean that the patient has cancer—they may be experiencing another disease or condition. However, if the patient *does* have cancer, there *will* be a blockage on the spinal column, because each vertebra controls a related internal organ's energy, or impulse function.

For example, when we find that T4 has a blockage, it does not mean the patient has breast or skin cancer, but if the patient has breast cancer or skin cancer, we can easily find the blockage in the T4 area.

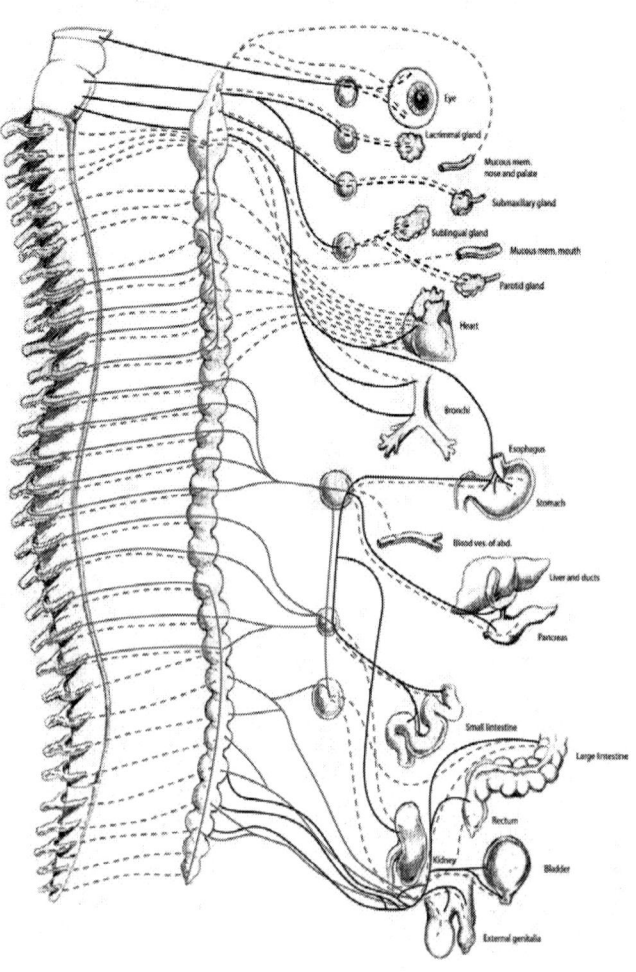

The Nervous System's Function

Let's consider the function of the nervous system. The message-passing network of the nervous system can be seen and detected in Western medical study. It passes impulses in either of two ways: by chemical synapse or by electrical synapse. The chemical synapse causes the chemical function in the body, and, of course, the electrical synapse causes the electrical function. However, in practice, we cannot separate these two.

Chemical synapses are specialized junctions through which neurons signal to each other and to non-neuronal cells (such as those in muscles or glands). Chemical synapses allow neurons to form circuits within the central nervous system and are crucial to the biological computations which are the basis of perception and thought. They allow the nervous system to connect to and control other systems of the body.

Compared to chemical synapses, electrical synapses are much faster at passing biosignals. Electrical synapses are often found in neural systems which require the fastest possible response, such as defensive reflexes and athletic movement. An important characteristic of electrical synapses is that they are mainly bidirectional, In other words, they allow impulse transmission in either direction, although some gap junctions do allow for communication in only one direction.

A quick example: hormones

In Western medical practice, chemical pills or drugs are used for hormone replacement, but many cause side effects. When one type of hormone is corrected, it may cause another hormone to go out of balance, and it is unfortunate that no interest is shown in using bioelectrical balance to bring hormone function back to normal.

In Eastern medicine, herbs or diet are used to correct hormone imbalance, but these are considered chemical sources for healing. Yet, Eastern medicine also uses mechanical, or physical, methods such as acupuncture, Tui Na, cupping, and other techniques to stimulate the meridian or acupuncture point to balance hormone problems.

Through medical testing, it is easy to determine hormone levels, but discovering which nerve triggers hormone activity is impossible—modern medical practice does not have a method or the knowledge to check nerves for a hormone trigger.

The Brain's Role

The brain is made of three main parts: the forebrain, midbrain, and hindbrain. The spinal cord and the brain work together. When we stimulate the brain, its impulse signal can pass to the spinal cord. Likewise, if we stimulate the spinal cord, the brain can receive the signal.

The brain system does not have nerves, but very rich blood vessels, and its job is to control nerve movement and function. So the brain does not have any blockage from the nervous system, but its problem may come from the blood circulation.

Though the brain is only 2% of the size of the whole body, it needs 20% of the blood circulation from the body. To keep the brain in good condition and functioning well, we must keep blood flowing freely from the two major arteries from the neck, the vertebral and common carotid arteries.

Human Cells as Miniature Batteries

The cell is the smallest unit of the body, and each cell has a life force. In fact, each individual cell is a 'battery' or capacitor that carries bioelectricity, which controls the function of that cell. The chemical material forms the cell and the structure of the cell stores bioelectricity.

Each cell has both a chemical and an electrical function, and each requires a chemical and electrical source for survival. In the medical world, people tend to favor the chemical function and chemical reaction of the cells. They separate the chemical function from the electrical function, or ignore the electrical function altogether.

A battery contains electrochemical cells that convert its stored chemical energy to electrical energy. When connected to a generator, a low battery can receive electrical charges from the generator and rebuild its stored energy. The body's cells have the same needs—they require the charge of bioelectricity to function normally. If a cell is experiencing a low voltage of bioelectricity and cannot be re-charged, it will not survive long.

When an auto mechanic checks a car battery, the first thing he does is check the voltage. However, when a medical expert checks cells, he tends to pay no attention to the voltage of those cells. Instead, his attention focuses on the cells' biochemistry.

The human body's 'batteries' need to stay charged and store bioelectricity. The blood supplies oxygen to the cell, but the nervous system triggers the function of the cell. Each organ's movement is controlled by its own nerve. The internal organ's impulse derives from the autonomic nervous system, which is formed by the sympathetic and parasympathetic nerves. When one of these nerves has a high resistance, it may interrupt the functioning of the organ or tissue. This, of course, can cause a cell problem as well.

Biochemistry vs Bioelectricity

In Tong Ren Healing, we accept that the chemical function of cells is important, but we realize that the electrical function is equally important. Because cells function as batteries, we need to understand both the chemical and electrical sides of the battery. If we do not pay attention to the bioelectricity in a cell, it is like a dead car battery—normal in physical structure, but without any electrical power!

It is no joke that many medical experts have never even heard about bioelectricity in the body. Some even deny its existence. But no one can deny that the human body produces electrical impulses. In the study of anatomy, it is known that both a chemical synapse and an electrical synapse control nerve function.

Based on what they choose to research, Western medicine focuses its attention on the chemical synapse. Untold amounts of money are invested into this research. I feel they should set aside even 1% of their budgets to research the neglected area of healing with bioelectricity. Indeed, this area of study is neglected, not because of a lack of funds, but because researchers feel that the concept of bioelectricity is too 'crazy' to pursue. I'm sure you know of Ph.D.'s in biology and biochemistry, but when was the last time you heard about someone getting a Ph.D. in bioelectricity?

Applying Ohm's Law to Human Bioelectricity

To understand the bioelectricity in our bodies, we can apply the principle of Ohm's law (**I =V/R**) to the nerve impulse or bioelectricity. According to this law, the conductor in the body is the nerve that passes a current of bioelectricity. The current (I) influences organ function. But what is the voltage (V)?

If we want the cells or organs to have higher current, we must lower the resistance from the nerve or raise the voltage from the brain. But how can we raise the voltage coming from the brain? Good question. We know that the voltage should come from the brain since all impulses come from the brain, but even our advanced medicine does not fully understand how the human brain functions and therefore we do not know where bioelectricity in the brain comes from.

So, where does bioelectricity come from? Traditional Chinese Medicine has an answer to this question: TCM believes that the Chi originates from the top of the head, called the Bai Hui point (GV20). Bai Hui in Chinese means, "hundred yang chi gather." This comes from years of healing experience rather than from scientific study.

Beyond Basic Anatomy: The Dantian and Shu Points

TCM believes that a newborn baby has a lot of Chi because its Dantian is filled with Chi, and because a baby breathes from the lower abdomen. When people get older, their Dantian weakens, and therefore it has less Chi. This causes breathing to become more shallow and causes shortness of breath. When people get old, their breathing originates in their chest, and when people are near death, breathing is from the throat, not the chest or abdomen. So TCM believes that if one desires longevity, they must have a strong Dantian for storage of more Chi.

In the West, it is believed that death occurs when the heart or brain stops functioning. In TCM, the meaning of death is when the person's Dantian has no more Chi. TCM believes if the Dantian is always kept full of Chi, it is a way to heal or prevent disease.

What is the Dantian?

Dantian is described as an important focal point for internal meditative techniques and refers specifically to the physical center of gravity. It is located in the abdomen about three finger widths below and two finger widths behind the navel.

The location of the Dantian is controversial in TCM. Some believe it is located four fingers below the navel. Acupuncture systems vary as well. Some say the Dantian is at CV4 and others believe it is at CV6.

In China, many practices have been developed to strengthen the Dantian, such as Tai Chi Chuan, Chi Gong, and many different breathing techniques. Other methods include the use of herbs or diet, moxibustion, acupuncture, as well as internal or external exercises. Taoist and Buddhist teachers often instruct their students to center their mind in the Dantian. Chinese martial arts require one to build up their Dantian so they can have the strength to break through stone or chop wood with their bare hand or head. Yet, the major practice is based on controlling one's breathing with the mind.

According to TCM, there are three different Dantian locations: the Upper Dantian, Middle Dantian, and Lower Dantian. The **Upper Dantian** is located on the third eye area, which is called Yintang in Chinese. It controls the mind's focus and emotion. The **Middle Dantian** is located on the chest, in the area between the two nipples (acupuncture point CV17). This area is for physical breathing. The **Lower Dantian** is on the CV4 or CV6 area—its function is to store Chi.

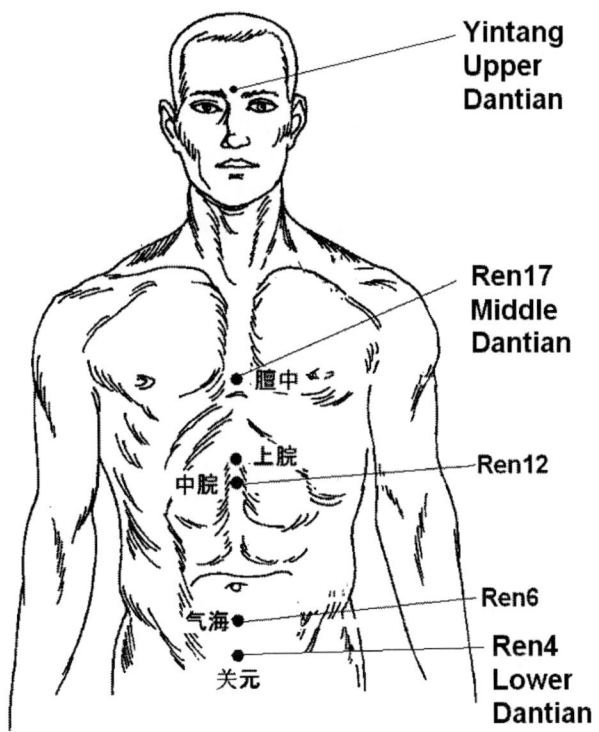

Triple Dantian Point Chart

In ancient times, there was no knowledge of the phrenic nerve, but everyone knew that air was important to life. TCM cannot understand the phrenic nerve and the breathing function, but now that we have much medical knowledge, we can use the phrenic nerve system to explain the whole Dantian theory.

To stay healthy, you must keep your Dantian in good condition. Now we can easily say that if one wants to stay healthy, one must have good oxygen levels, which means keeping the phrenic nerve free.

TCM believes that any disease is caused by the blood or Chi being out of balance. Now, we can put the phrenic nerve system into the Dantian system for healing or energy practice.

Meridians are the Highway for *Chi*

Traditional Chinese Medicine (TCM) believes that oxygen is a very important part of our life force, and have given it the name **Chi**. TCM developed the practice of Chi Gong which includes techniques focused on breathing to increase the body's oxygen capacity. Many ancient energy practices utilize breathing techniques to increase the intake of air and the capacity of the lungs. All cells and organs need oxygen in order to function, and inhaling brings oxygen into the body. This oxygen is then transported by the blood to nourish cells. But when the cells carry a low level of oxygen, it can cause many forms of disease.

In TCM theory, the **meridians** are pathways for the circulation of Chi (there are fourteen of them in the human body), and each internal organ has its own. Each meridian has many energy points, and each organ has its own energy point as well.

The bladder meridian, for instance, which consists of 67 meridian points, is the longest. The bladder meridian starts from the head in the inner corner of eye area where the inner canthus is located and ascends to the forehead, joining the governing vessel meridian (GV20) at the vertex where a branch goes to the temple. The straight portion enters and communicates with the brain. It emerges and bifurcates to descend along the posterior aspect of the neck. It runs down along the back and enters the body cavity at the lumbar region, connecting with the kidney and joining the bladder.

The lumbar branch descends through the gluteal region and ends in the popliteal fossa. The branch from the neck runs down the back and reunites in the popliteal fossa, descending down the leg to the lateral side of the little toe.

An organ's yang energy point in TCM is called the **Shu point**; the yin energy point is called the Mu point. For example, the lung's energy point is called the Lung Shu, the heart has the Heart Shu, and so on.

The sympathetic nerves, which run from the spinal cord, work together with the parasympathetic nerves. For example, the heart's movement is controlled by the sympathetic and parasympathetic nerve, since one nerve speeds up the heart rate while the other slows it down. TCM designates the energy source point on the back, beside the spinal column. This energy source point is called the Shu point. Each internal organ has its own Shu point, such as the liver Shu, heart Shu, or lung Shu.

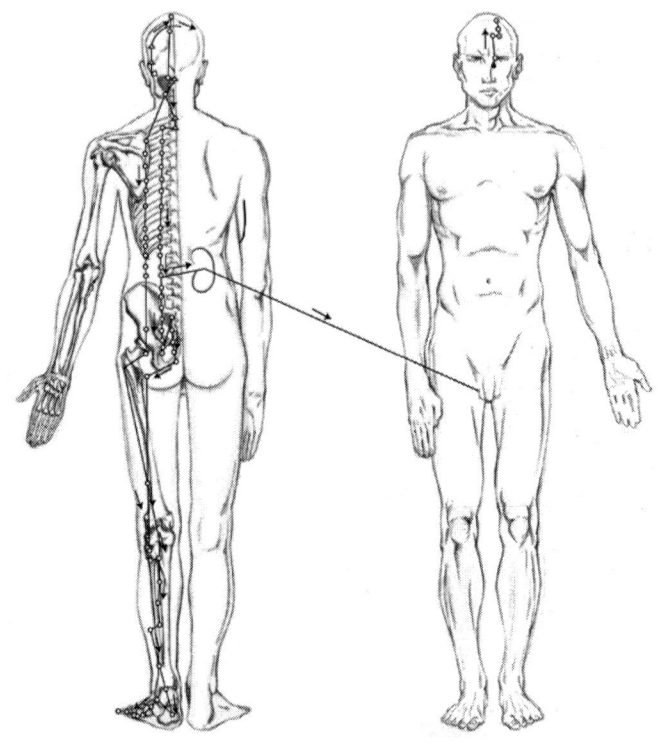

Track of Bladder Meridian

Ancient TCM did not know anything about the sympathetic nerves, but through their experience, they could determine that the energy point was in the back.

By TCM theory, if we stimulate the bladder meridian points on the head area, then it may affect the Chi running to the spinal column and the toe. By Western medical theory, if the brain gets stimulated, its impulse may follow the spinal cord down to the leg and the toe, also.

Each organ's Shu point is near the spinal column, on the bladder meridian and close to the sympathetic nerve. If we use scientific knowledge to understand the sympathetic nerve, then it is easy to understand the function of the Shu points.

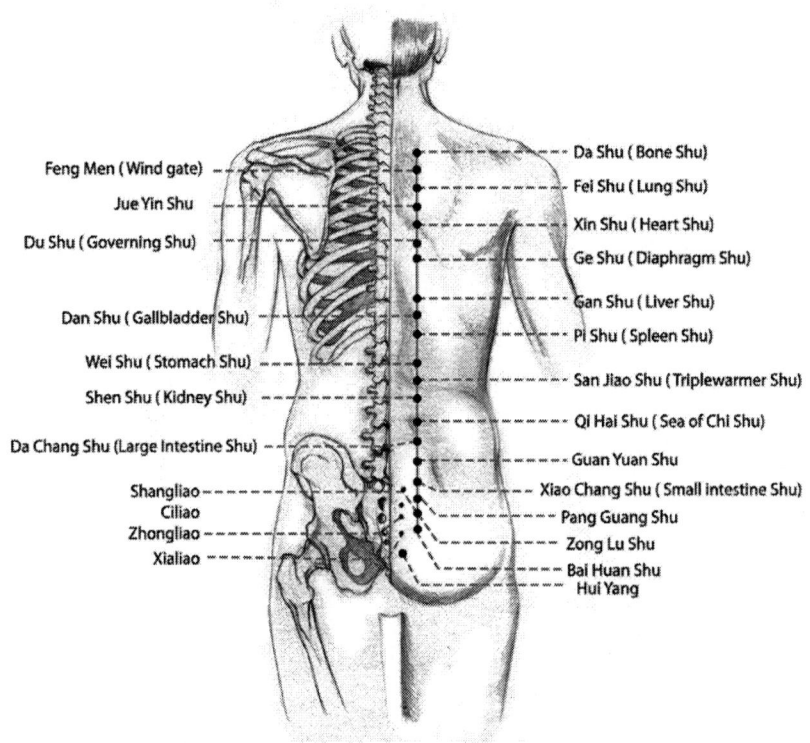

Shu Point on the back's Bladder Meridian

Each vertebral column has a Shu point on the bladder meridian. Yet, closer to the spinal column, we have the Hua Tuo Jia Ji points, which were developed almost two thousand years ago in *Three Warring States* by Dr. Hua Tuo (145 - 208 AC).

Dr. Hua Tuo's development—also called *Huatuojiaji* in Chinese—means "next to the spinal column." Huatuojiaji does not belong to any particular meridian—they are simply extra points located between the bladder meridian and the governing vessel meridian (which is closer to the spinal cord).

In the Tom Tam Healing System, we use the Huatuojiaji points more than the Shu points, because we most often find blockages there. The healing meaning of Huatuojiaji points are confusing, and much of the ancient information has been lost. But the Tom Tam Healing System, through study and healing experiences with patients, has compiled a new annotation with the Huatuojiaji points.

The bladder meridian is located on the right and left sides of the back and each Shu point on the left and right side are the same. For instance, on both the right and left sides of T9 on the bladder meridian is the Liver Shu.

In my practice, I do not follow the back Shu points from the TCM bladder meridian and have updated the lost Huatuojiaji points along the lines of common sense and anatomy. In the study of anatomy, the left and right brain are not the same, so, logically, the left and right parts of the nervous system should not be the same.

San Jiao

Another meridian system is called **San Jiao**, also referred to as the *Triple Heater*, *Triple Warmer* (or *Three Warmers*), and *Triple Burner*. Triple Warmer references can be found in the oldest Chinese medical textbook, the *Yellow Emperor's Inner Canon*, or *Huang Di Nei Jing*.

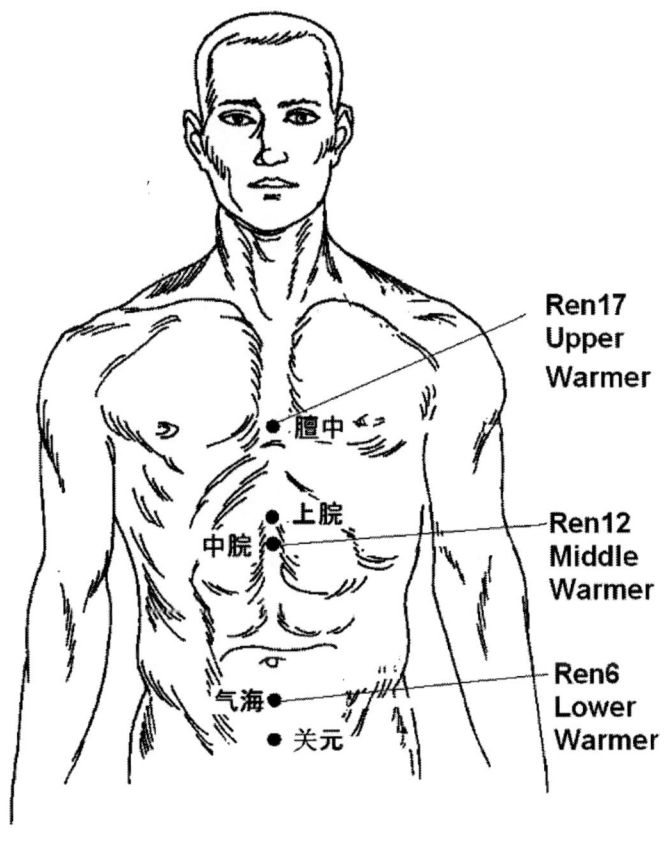

Triple Warmer Point Chart

Healing Cancer with the Nervous System

华佗夾脊新註简图
New Annotation of Huatuojiaji Points

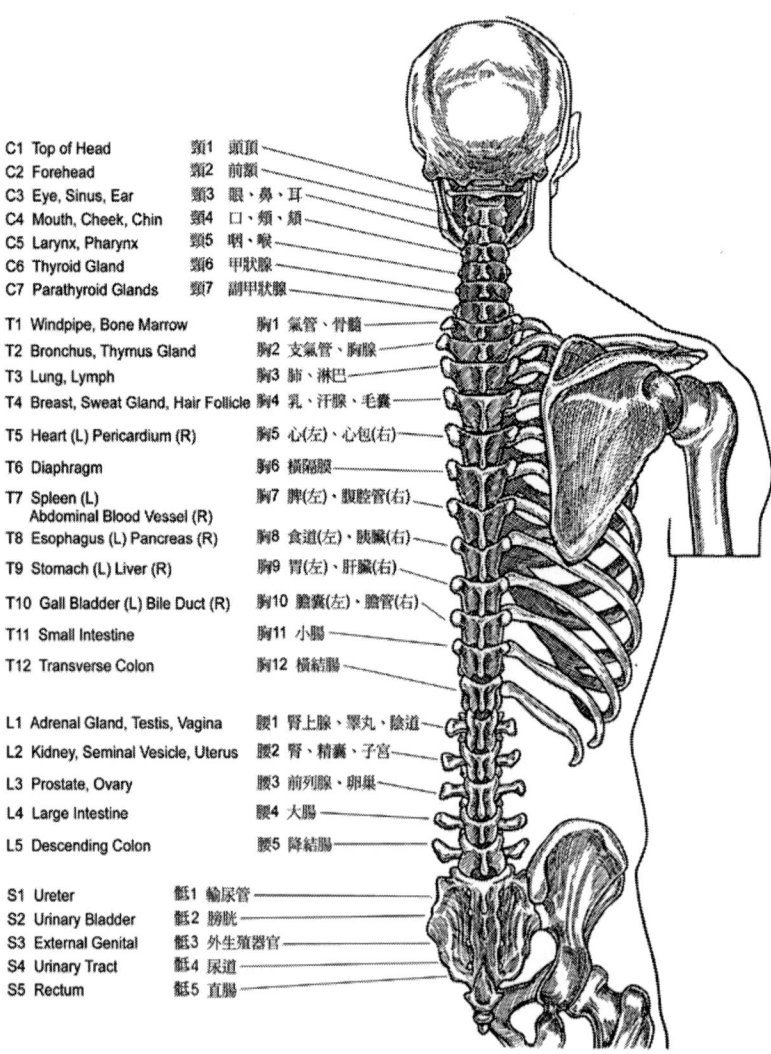

C1	Top of Head	頸1	頭頂
C2	Forehead	頸2	前額
C3	Eye, Sinus, Ear	頸3	眼、鼻、耳
C4	Mouth, Cheek, Chin	頸4	口、頰、頦
C5	Larynx, Pharynx	頸5	咽、喉
C6	Thyroid Gland	頸6	甲狀腺
C7	Parathyroid Glands	頸7	副甲狀腺
T1	Windpipe, Bone Marrow	胸1	氣管、骨髓
T2	Bronchus, Thymus Gland	胸2	支氣管、胸腺
T3	Lung, Lymph	胸3	肺、淋巴
T4	Breast, Sweat Gland, Hair Follicle	胸4	乳、汗腺、毛囊
T5	Heart (L) Pericardium (R)	胸5	心(左)、心包(右)
T6	Diaphragm	胸6	橫隔膜
T7	Spleen (L) Abdominal Blood Vessel (R)	胸7	脾(左)、腹腔管(右)
T8	Esophagus (L) Pancreas (R)	胸8	食道(左)、胰臟(右)
T9	Stomach (L) Liver (R)	胸9	胃(左)、肝臟(右)
T10	Gall Bladder (L) Bile Duct (R)	胸10	膽囊(左)、膽管(右)
T11	Small Intestine	胸11	小腸
T12	Transverse Colon	胸12	橫結腸
L1	Adrenal Gland, Testis, Vagina	腰1	腎上腺、睾丸、陰道
L2	Kidney, Seminal Vesicle, Uterus	腰2	腎、精囊、子宮
L3	Prostate, Ovary	腰3	前列腺、卵巢
L4	Large Intestine	腰4	大腸
L5	Descending Colon	腰5	降結腸
S1	Ureter	骶1	輸尿管
S2	Urinary Bladder	骶2	膀胱
S3	External Genital	骶3	外生殖器官
S4	Urinary Tract	骶4	尿道
S5	Rectum	骶5	直腸

Triple Warmers include the upper, middle, and lower warmers. The Triple Warmer's function is to regulate all internal organ connections and functions. This theory is abstract and confuses many experts. Even in TCM, there is still debate regarding the meaning of the Triple Warmer and the location of its meridian track. But if we use the vagus nerve system, it is easy to understand the Triple Warmers.

The Great Plexuses of the Sympathetic System are aggregations of nerves and ganglia, situated in the thoracic, abdominal, and pelvic cavities (which are the cardiac, celiac, and hypogastric plexuses). These plexuses consist not only of sympathetic fibers derived from the ganglia, but of fibers from the medulla spinalis, which communicate through the white rami. The plexus branches flow to the thoracic, abdominal, and pelvic viscera.

Ancient TCM did not have knowledge about the parasympathetic nerve or the great plexuses. However, from the description of the Triple Warmer meridian, we can deduce that the Upper Warmer should be the cardiac plexus, the Middle Warmer should be the celiac plexus, and the Lower Warmer should be the hypogastric plexus.

In healing practice, we have difficulty treating the Great Plexuses of the Sympathetic System because they are so well protected. The most common

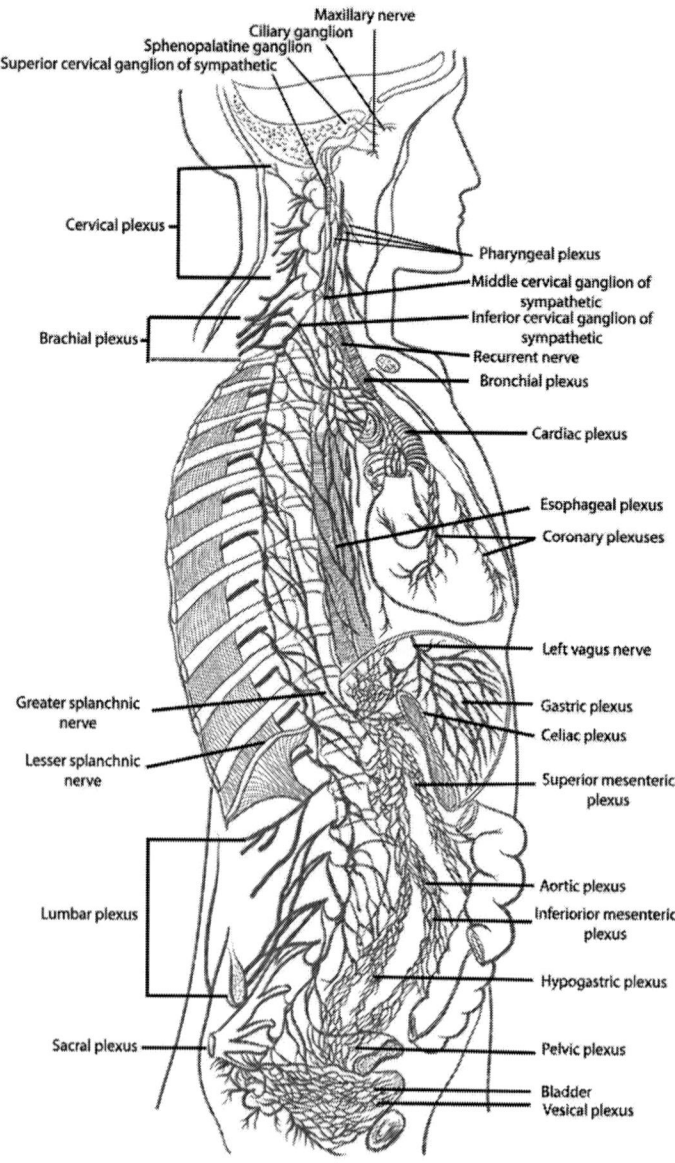

Vagus Nerve

blockage point, which can be found on the Large Intestine Meridian, is called Futu (LI18). The sympathetic nerves run alongside the spinal column and can easily become pinched by poor spinal posture, overuse, injury, or muscle tension in the back. The autonomic nervous system must be kept in good condition in order to maintain normal bio-current to the organs.

The vagus nerve passes along the neck area under LI18. It is one of the brain's cranial nerves, originating at the brain stem and passing down to the neck, then to the chest cavity and connecting to each internal organ. The vagus nerve is well protected within the chest cavity, which means that most often the blockage of this nerve originates in the neck area, due to muscle tension from overuse, poor posture, or injury.

LI18 is located near the common carotid artery. When we use acupuncture or Tui Na to stimulate LI18, we must pay attention to avoid the common carotid artery.

Traditional Chinese Medicine believes that all Shu points are located on the bladder meridian on the back, but in the Tom Tam Healing System, the energy points are located just beside the spinal column, which are called the Hua Tuo Jia Ji points. These points do not belong to any meridians from the body, but simply to a nerve from the spinal cord.

TCM believes that when the Shu point becomes blocked, it may cause Chi stagnation in a particular organ. For example, when the liver has a problem, the blockage may show on the right side of the spinal column on T9. According to the Tom Tam Healing System, when an organ has a problem, we can find the point of blockage (or Ouch point) beside the spinal column. Each energy source point beside the spinal column has its own organ's connection. For example, with breast cancer we find the blockage on T4; with lung cancer, it is beside T3; and in prostate and ovarian cancers, the blockage is beside L3.

Looking Deeper at the Bladder Meridians

TCM theory believes that the bladder meridians are located on both sides of the body. The bladder meridians run along the same side of the body, meaning the left bladder meridian runs in the left side of the body, and the right bladder meridian runs in the right side of the body. However, from anatomy study, we find that the left side of the brain controls the right side of the body and vice versa.

Similarly, the motor cortex in the right side of the brain controls movement in the left side of the body. When a stroke occurs in the right side of the brain, it may cause the left side of the patient's body to lose movement and function. And from modern anatomy, we know that stimulating the left side of the brain results in an impulse that follows the right side of the spinal cord.

This knowledge of human anatomy contradicts the TCM belief that the meridians control the same side of the body. In fact, in my practice of acupuncture, when we put the needle on the left side of the skull, the Chi or impulse will follow on the right side of the body.

In TCM theory, the bladder meridian in BL10, located in the neck area, is divided into two tracks, then continues down the spinal column. I believe the bladder meridian in BL10 crosses the spinal column, switching to the other side of BL9. This makes more sense and a better match with Western medical theory. Why do TCM practitioners think in this way?

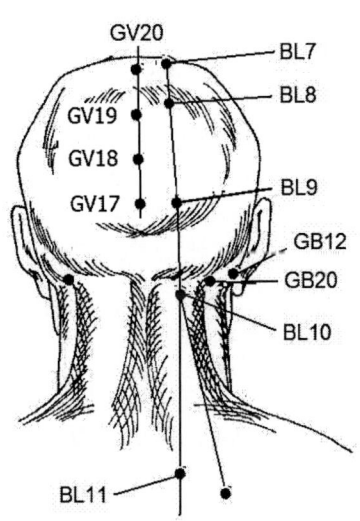

These skull bladder meridian points may not be blockage points, but they can help blockages in other areas. When we insert needles or use other techniques to stimulate these points, most people feel Chi running down their back, arms, and legs. It means that the function of these points can release tension from the muscle.

In the Tom Tam Healing System, we believe many blockages maybe caused by muscular tension. When the tension is released, the nerve resistor should drop down. If resistance drops, it causes the bio-current to increase. Interestingly, when the skull acupuncture point is stimulated, it may raise the voltage in a particular part of the brain, which can improve the function of the central nervous system.

Where and How Did the Meridian System Originate?

To understand the meridian system, we must understand how the meridians were discovered in ancient China. The healing practice for patients began with therapeutic touch or massage, which the Chinese call **Tui Na** (or, as some in the West call it, acupressure). In ancient China, through cumulative clinical treatments, healers confirmed that particular spots in the body directly affected healing results. Through repeated empirical practice in healing, Chinese practitioners discovered more and more points that were effective in healing a variety of illnesses. Early on, some healers realized that arranging these healing points in a line aided teaching and memorization.

In addition, ancient China had highly developed energy practices, which are now called Chi Gong or Dao Yin. During this energy practice, healers felt the energy on particular points of the body and felt how the energy followed a line to a particular organ.

This track line along which Chi moves is called the meridian. When the line produced a sensation of heat, tingling, heaviness, or numbness and related it to a specific organ, ancient practitioners conferred the terminus organ's name as the name for that meridian, (e.g., the Heart meridian, Stomach meridian, etc.).

Over the centuries, as this system was developed, many more energy points were discovered. Other healing systems are finding new energy points for healing as well. TCM developed twelve meridians which connected to twelve organs, and have two main meridians to balance the yin and yang energy. These fourteen meridians are also linked via other connecting meridians. Therefore, TCM believes that the whole body is a unit connected by meridians, and when these are transporting signals freely, with no blockages at the acupuncture points, then Chi moves freely and the organs function normally.

In fact, even in Western anatomy and physiology, medical experts have found many energy points useful to their practice, including Dermatome locations which are taught in medical school. For example, when people experience pain anywhere in their body, the symptoms may be referred from the back where the spinal nerves or spinal cord is blocked. According to the Tom Tam Healing System, the Dermatome locations information chart can be used to heal cancer as well.

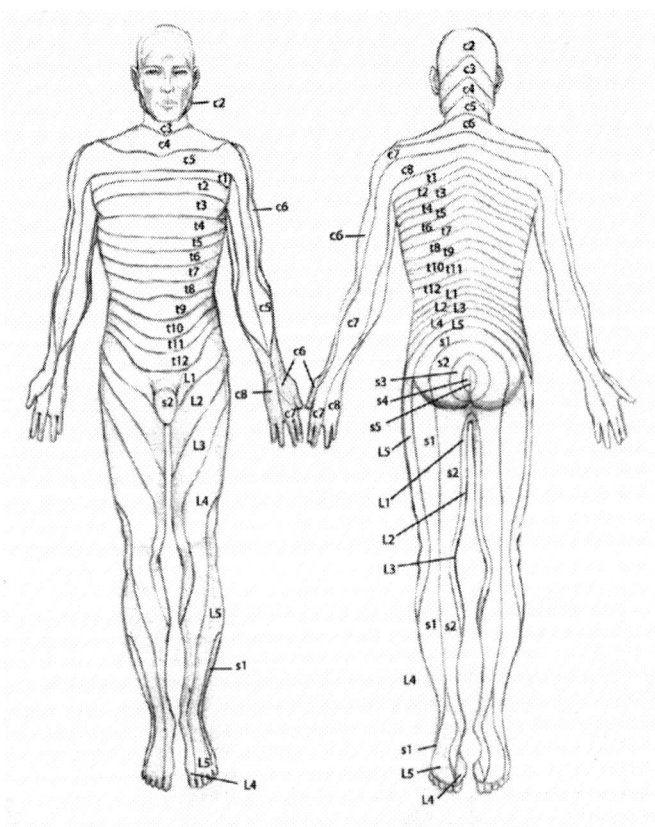

Dermatome Locations

Western medical training utilizes the referred pain theory, sometimes referred to as reflective pain. When pain is felt in one area of the body, it does not always represent where the cause of the problem is actually located—the pain may be 'referred' there from another area. For example, pain produced by a heart attack may feel as if it is coming from the arm because sensory information from both the heart and the arm converge on the same nerve pathways in the spinal cord.

Yet, in acupuncture theory, more than two thousand years ago, healers already knew that to heal a heart problem, including heart attack and angina, the practitioner could use P6 (Pericardium 6) or P7 (Pericardium 7), which are the meridian points on the arm. Here is the irony: Western medicine is well versed in many referred pain points that relate to a problem in a particular organ, yet it uses this knowledge only in extremely limited ways: for diagnosis, but not for healing!

The West discovered the biology of 'trigger' points. Many chiropractors and massage therapists find the model useful in practice, but the medical community at large has not embraced trigger point therapy. The trigger point is an area or point that feels painful, which in TCM is called the Ouch point (the names are different, but the meanings are the same).

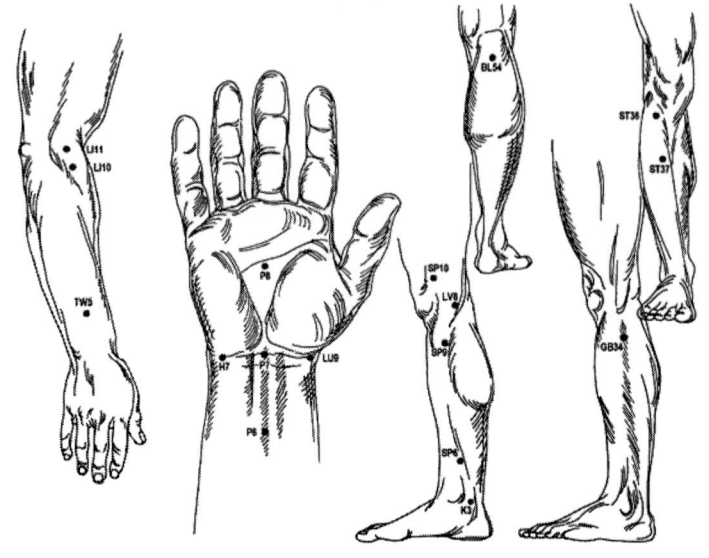

P6 and P7 can heal heart problems

When the Chinese discovered the Ouch point, they used their own methods to physically stimulate this point, such as with acupuncture, moxa, Tui Na, or another method to release the pain. An Ouch point can be located anywhere within the body.

In Western medicine, reflective pain is used only for diagnosis. When a doctor determines the reflective pain area, his technique for healing is most often prescribing medication to mask the pain or performing surgery.

For example, for common problems like lower back pain or migraine headaches, the West recommends medication for healing. Yet, they do not consider a protocol in their practice that would address the reflective pain or energy point, which can increase the range of healing.

It is not important that Western medical practice will not accept the concept of the meridian system. What *is* important is understanding and using energy points in the body, or the reflective points, in their own way. Without a doubt, as Eastern medicine has shown, these energy points or meridian points can heal sickness when properly stimulated. Though the West also denies the efficacy of acupuncture and other methods of stimulation, yet, in fact, any mechanical, physical, or electrical stimulation holds the potential to initiate a reaction within the body which may trigger healing.

When we understand the meaning of meridians, we can compare the meridian system with the nervous system. When a nerve becomes blocked from a pinch, anesthesia, injury, or when the patient experiences a stroke, sensations or feelings of moving Chi are not detectable—this means that Chi movement cannot be separated from the nervous system.

If we use the nervous system to explain the meridians, we never can compare them. However, if we use multi-nervous systems to understand the meridians, it is much easier to draw a parallel. For example, the Large Intestine meridian begins at the tip of the index finger, takes a particular path up the arm to the highest point of the shoulder, runs along the cervical vertebrae and collarbone before connecting to the lung and finally to the diaphragm, large intestine, and lower abdomen.

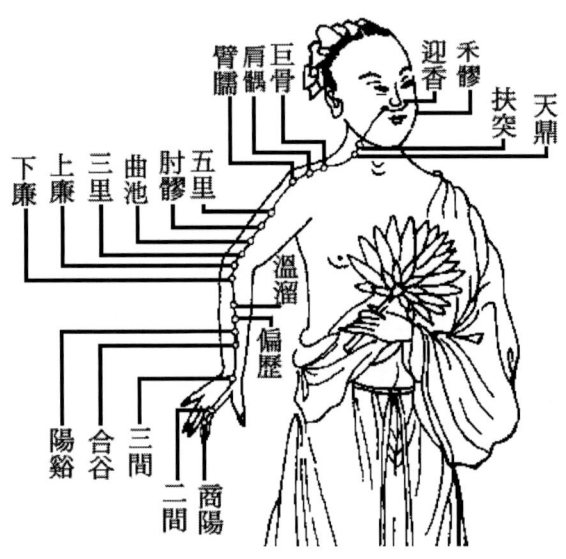

Meridian points of the Large Intestine

The Large Intestine meridian running from the index finger to the shoulder and neck is easy to understand because the radial nerve is located at the neck where the brachial plexus runs down to the finger. However, energy running to the face is difficult to understand when looking at the radial nerve.

How does the Large Intestine meridian enter the face? The answer lies in the fact that the facial artery and facial nerve run to this area, affecting blood circulation to the face—and we know that meridians affect blood circulation in addition to Chi movement.

The meridian point ST12 is found around the subclavian artery area, which runs to the hand for blood circulation. When we stimulate LI4, it means the stimulation can create a signal following the radial nerve upward to C5 (the location of the brachial plexus). When C5 receives the signal from LI4, it may affect the facial artery and facial nerve, taking the signal to the facial area.

LI4 is a point very often used for any style of acupuncture and acupressure. But in the Tom Tam Healing System, LI4 is a seldom-used point; instead, ST12 or other points are used. ST12 can release tension in the neck and scapular directly. TCM belief is that the Chi's circulation needs the blood's nourishment. ST12 is close to the subclavian artery that sends the blood to nourish the LI4 point area.

The concept of the Large Intestine meridian running to the face and neck is easy to accept and understand. However, the question arises about its track from the neck down to the lung and large intestine. Stimulation of LI4, which is on the thumb area, can affect the movement affect the large intestine or abdominal area.

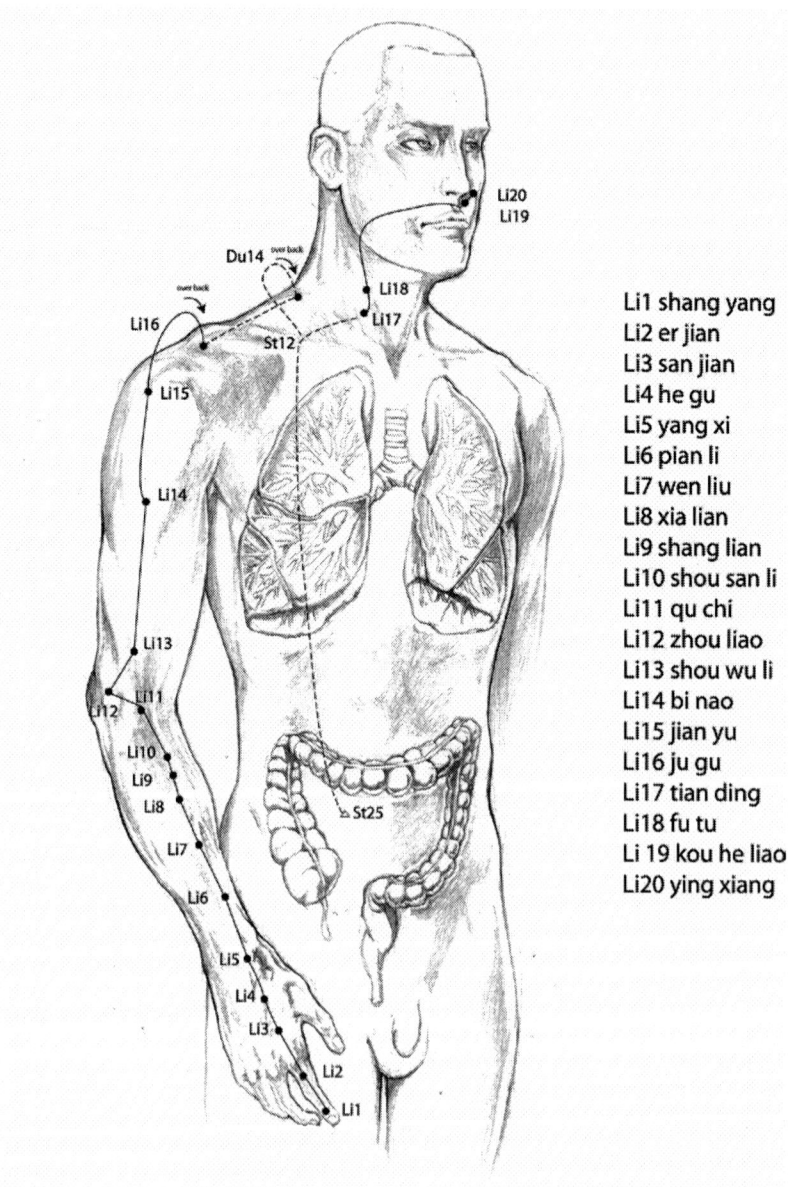

The Chi track runs of Large Intestine Meridian

So far, no one can explain this phenomenon. Yet, with the Tom Tam Healing System, it is easy to understand this, because when LI4 is stimulated, the impulse can affect the neck area. In the neck area, C5 is the location of both the radial nerve and the phrenic nerve. The phrenic nerve runs from C5 toward the lung and lower abdomen and then to the diaphragm.

The Large Intestine point Qishe (LI18) is located at the vagus nerve area on the neck beside the ST11 point that connects to all internal organs. So, to understand the Large Intestine meridian, we should combine the information we have about the radial nerve, subclavian artery, facial artery, facial nerve, phrenic nerve and vagus nerve, and then we can easily understand the theory of meridians.

TCM theory believes that when Chi is running, then blood is circulating well, so the feeling of Chi is included with the feeling of blood flow. For instance, during a Chi Gong treatment or Tong Ren healing, some people feel heat or warmth on the face or palm, which is the blood carrying oxygen and raising the metabolism function. Sometimes people may feel tingling, which is the movement of bioelectricity. Many people can feel their chest open and receive more oxygen, which are the lung and phrenic nerves functioning. Therefore, when considering meridians, do not limit their function to moving Chi alone, consider blood circulation as well.

Different Viewpoints on Meridians and the Nervous System

It is common knowledge that at the crux of healing is the ability to prove a healing concept with scientific results. Yet, there is a vast difference between the concepts adopted in the West and East, in addition to traditional medicine, alternative medicine, and complementary medicine—each embraces its own theory.

Western medicine is based on modern scientific study, but lacks healing experience. The healing methods of conventional medicine follow a limited path. Medicine from the East still follows the traditional method, even when it is combined with Western medicine. Every medical theory—Western, Eastern, traditional, alternative, or even complementary—claims that its approach represents 'science' and true healing. This controversy is comparable to that of religion—the debate never ends.

The difference between Western and Eastern medicine is in the theory and healing method of meridians. Meridians cannot be seen nor detected by any modern high-tech equipment, and Western practitioners resist believing in anything that it cannot see with their equipment or through laboratory examination. On the other hand, TCM practitioners do not accept the West's belief that denies the existence of meridians. Lately, in China some scientists and doctors have tried to unite the Western and Eastern medical philosophies, yet, it is not an easy job, because Chinese scientific study cannot tangibly prove its theory of the nerve system and meridians. So, is there an effective way to marry these two systems?

There is no doubt that acupuncture or meridian stimulation relate to nervous system stimulation, despite the fact that Western medicine does not accept it. Choosing a healing strategy should follow common sense: if the problem stems from a chemical function, use chemicals to balance and heal the illness, but if the problem relates to bioelectrical dysfunction, chemicals will not help.

Western medicine has expansive knowledge about the nervous system, but does not respect the concept of energy points nor shows interest in learning about how to use them for healing. In addition, many medical experts laugh at or criticize acupuncture and the concept of meridians.

It is sad that they criticize other healing systems—they are missing an entire body of knowledge that could enhance their own system. To treat the nerve function problems, we must have nervous system points just as TCM has acupuncture points. Only then can the Western medical system complete its healing system, including the biochemical and bioelectrical functions.

Western medicine tries to find the blockage in the nerve functionally, with modern equipment. They test the nerve conductivity, often in the case of the sciatic nerve. In some cases after this test the pain can be released, as it often is in acupuncture, because the electric probe provides a form of stimulation. However, this healing response may not be acknowledged.

Through X-ray and MRI equipment nerve problems can be identified. Even many chiropractors use x-ray equipment in their offices. Undoubtedly, an X-ray and an MRI can find a pinched nerve, however, many nerve problems will never show up with the use of any machine; they are only detectable by the touch of a skilled practitioner's hand.

It is strange that medical practitioners prefer to depend on high-tech equipment than on touching their patients. Nerves are not only pinched by bones or discs, but they can be blocked by soft tissue or muscular tension as well.

When a nerve is inflamed, it may cause the nerve to malfunction. Western healing developed many methods to stimulate the muscular or nervous system, however, these methods continue to show low healing rates. This is because they fail to consider the use of energy points. Stimulating the nervous system (and knowing the correct area(s) to stimulate) is crucial to healing nerve-related problems.

On the other hand, TCM does not refer to a nervous system or identify nerves (it refers only to the meridian system), but, from a long history of healing, it recognizes the function of energy points and locations. Through modern Chinese medical study, it was discovered that all acupuncture points are located on the nerves or around the nerve areas and vessels. This means that when we stimulate the acupuncture points, the nervous system is stimulated.

In TCM when a point or nerve is anesthetized, Chi cannot pass and there is no Chi sensation. In the same respect, in the case of an injured nerve or a stroke, the patient will not feel Chi movement.

Does 'Nervous System' = 'Meridian System'?

The nervous system is developed from scientific study, and the meridian system is developed from the healing experience of TCM. So, is the meridian system equal to the nervous system? No one has yet answered this question. Too many medical experts are quick to give an easy answer: that meridians do not exist (but this is based on their own inability to conceptualize the meridians due to their lack of training and clinical experience).

The worst "scientists" call the meridian theory 'quack' medicine. These scientists are called the Skeptics. They deny not only meridians, but the entire TCM healing system, including herbs and acupuncture. Skeptics have been active in America for a long time, but now they are appearing in China. The Chinese Skeptics want the government to stop all TCM practice in China, and to follow only the Western medical system. The argument about whether doctors should or should not continue TCM practice in China has been raging for the last 100 years.

Indeed, this type of extreme denial and denigration of other healing systems is an abnormal psychological problem, which is called Neophobia. This psychological problem is harmful to the health of society, because 'experts' mislead the public and disparage a medical system supported by thousands of years of clinical research while pushing their political agendas instead of scientifically studying the problem and the healing results experienced through TCM.

Free Radicals and the Kidney Meridian

The growth or mutation of cells within the body is a topic of great concern. It relates to the following four basic factors: oxygen, protein, growth hormone, and bioelectricity.

Oxygen is a requirement for survival in all forms of life. The Warburg Effect theorizes that after 48 hours of oxygen deprivation, normal cells can become cancerous. Because cancer cells thrive in an environment with low (or no) oxygen, the first items to consider in healing cancer are oxygen intake and blood circulation. The human body is an obligate aerobic organism whose cells require oxygen to oxidize or convert nutrients into the energy needed for normal cell functions. The level of oxygen within the body is affected by the intake during normal breathing and the transportation of that oxygen through arteries and veins to the organs.

Protein is important for normal cell growth. Therefore, a sound diet that includes quality sources of protein is imperative to ensure normal cell growth. Many people believe that a vegetarian diet can heal and prevent cancer, but this is a misconception. Medical studies show no difference in the cancer death rate between patients following a vegetarian diet and those on a diet which includes meat. Although a good diet can help the process of healing, it is not a major factor in curing cancer. In fact, as the body loses healthy cells during and after chemotherapy or radiation treatments, it needs protein to help form healthy cells. In my opinion, when cancer patients undergo the Big Three treatments, they should eat more protein and a high-calorie diet to build back their body's energy.

Everyone knows that cells need **growth hormone**, which is a major component of metabolism. If normal growth hormone is present, then cells can grow in a healthy way. In treating cancer, most doctors focus on the immune system, not on the metabolic system. It is widely accepted that the general treatment therapy for cancer patients is to kill their cancer cells. However, stopping cell mutation once it has begun is nearly impossible. It is important to create an environment in the body where mutation will not be triggered in the first place.

Each cell, like a battery, uses **bioelectricity** for normal cell functions. When the level of bioelectricity gets low or when the signal carried becomes negatively charged, those cells will stop functioning and growing normally. This is a logical factor to consider when studying cancer, but, sadly, researchers place their emphasis on biochemistry instead. Even those studying DNA focus on the structure and chemical form of the cell, not on the bioelectricity that the cell needs to function properly.

Free Radicals

At the University of Michigan in 1900, Moses Gomberg was the first to identify what are now called free radicals. In 1954, Denham Harmon proposed that free radicals were the cause of damage to macromolecules, known as "aging" or the aging process. Although there was an initial reluctance to accept his theory, the medical community has come to embrace his research and now focuses on how free radicals might be linked to healing cancers and degenerative diseases.

We know that radicals are necessary for normal body functions, but too many radicals can be harmful. The body needs to produce an immune response to clean out the excess free radicals.

Lately, Western medicine is giving considerable attention to the study of free radicals, called Free Radical Biology. Many experts believe that the study of free radicals is a revolution for modern medicine that can bring new hope for healing a wide range of diseases and conditions. It brings modern medicine into the age of bioelectronics, a discipline emerging from the merger of electronics and electrical engineering with biology, physics, chemistry, and materials science. It is the next generation of healthcare technology.

What are free radicals?

So, what are free radicals? Free radicals (also known as radicals) are atoms, molecules, or ions with unpaired electrons and, in general they are very chemically reactive. Ions can have a positive, negative, or zero charge. A radical that is missing an electron will have a positive charge. If it has an extra electron, it will have a negative charge.

Radicals perform several important functions in the human body. In fact, life cannot exist without some radicals in the body. Radicals naturally occur within the normal chemical reaction known as metabolism. Radicals control specific cellular functions, are a necessary part of chemical processes within the body, and serve as signal transducers. They are generated by the immune system that uses them as markers on foreign bodies or damaged tissues that the body can later remove.

The human body has two kinds of radicals, 95% of which are oxygen-free radicals and the remainder non-oxygen-free radicals. The oxygen free radicals react with oxygen molecules, taking an electron to complete their electron pair, but creating another radical in their wake.

Radical formation can be stimulated through external sources. These include stress, toxins in the environment, smoking, pesticides, air pollution, water pollution, and antibiotics in meat and dairy products. Because radicals are so chemically reactive, an excessive amount of radicals can damage DNA, resulting in mutations that alter the cell cycle. Cells can be injured, impairing cell function, resulting in cell death, degenerative diseases, and cancers. Thus, free radicals can be good and bad, depending on the situation.

For instance, oxygen is a fuel to fire, but in the presence of moisture, it can rust metal. In the body, too many radicals lead to the equivalent of the rusting of metal.

We know that biological functions in the human body have both a chemical and an electrical function. However, medical research focuses on the biological function in the chemical reaction, not on the electrical reaction. If only the chemical function is studied and understood, half of the body's function is being ignored.

To understand free radicals in the body, we must first understand the functions and reactions in our body. In the study of medicine, everyone knows that the body has two functions—biochemical and bioelectrical–and has two reactions—again, biochemical and bioelectrical.

The key question is: do free radicals belong to a biochemical or a bioelectrical *function*, or are they part of a biochemical or bioelectrical *reaction*? Research to date focuses on the *chemical* function and the *chemical* reaction. This is demonstrated by the many new drug therapies developed to combat free radicals.

Medical studies support the use of antioxidants as effective inhibitors against radicals. Pharmaceutical companies portray free radicals as thoroughly 'bad' and suggest that their drugs are required to eliminate them from our bodies. You get the impression that you must rid the body of radicals to experience good health. Many nutritionists advise their patients to avoid certain foods and take vitamins or minerals in their place—again, a *chemical* response to a problem within the body instead of the *bioelectrical* element.

In a single day, every cell in our body is attacked by a free radical an estimated 10,000 times while burning calories through the metabolic process. As we get older, the number of free radicals in our body naturally increases. Certain activities such as exercise and bodybuilding can also cause the body to produce more free radicals.

In fact, any process that stresses the body and abnormally increases the intake of oxygen can lead to an increase in free radicals.

Using semiconductor theory to understand free radicals

We know there are four different metallic conductors: the superconductor, conductor, semiconductor, and insulator. In the human body, we cannot physically have a superconductor, which has an electrical resistance of zero. Science tells us that, to date, humans have not been found to have zero electrical resistance. In fact, measurements show the human body has a voltage of less than 100 millivolts.

A human body with low resistance is acting as a conductor while one with high resistance is acting as a semiconductor. Semiconductors and human nerves pass electricity and bioelectricity in only one direction.

When an electron leaves the molecule, it is called a free electron. Semiconductor theory explains that when a molecule is triggered by an electrical signal, the electron may separate from the molecule.

Healing Cancer with the Nervous System

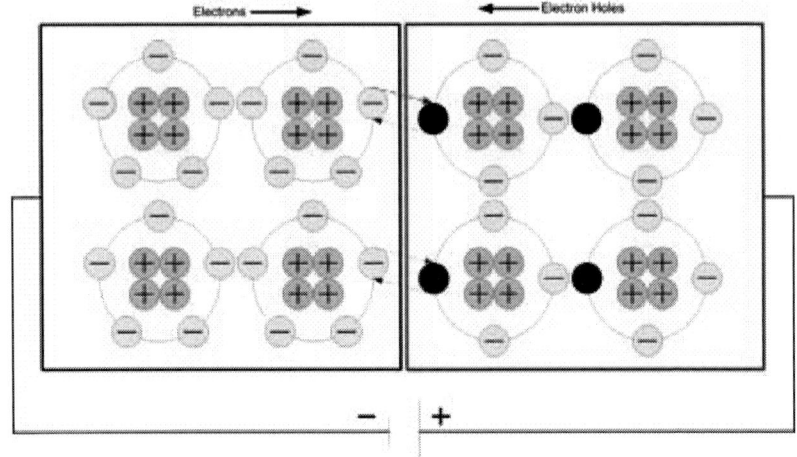

Oxygen free radical movement

At the atomic level, free electrons jump from one shell to another, filling nearby positive charge carriers or holes in the crystal structure of the semiconductor. In jumping, each electron leaves a hole behind for the next free electron to fill, creating a flow of electrons.

In the semiconductor, electron movement involves no chemical reaction, only an electrical one. From the study of biochemistry, we know that the free radical is the way oxygen passes energy (through bioelectricity) from molecule to molecule.

Electron Transport Chain theory tells us that as electrons are passed between electron donor molecules to electron receptor molecules. This is linked, by side biochemical reactions, to the passing of ions through the cell membrane. This transport mechanism is used to extract energy from nutrients (e.g. oxidation of sugars) and pass that energy into the cell.

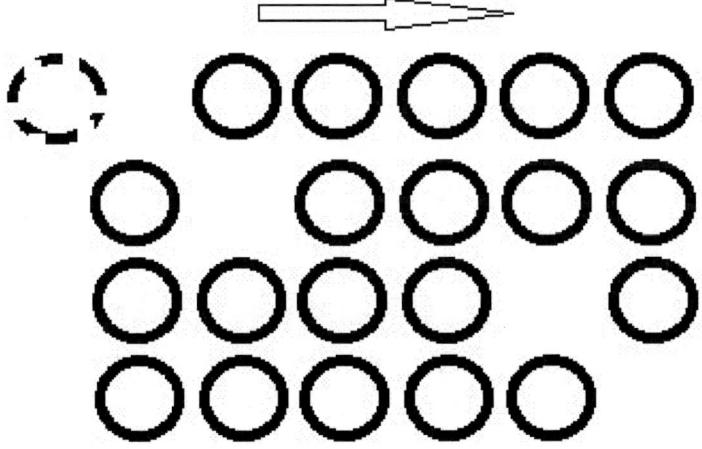

Electron Hole Movement in Semiconductors

When the number of free radicals within the body is out of balance, the body will become sick. Two things determine the extent, if any, of cell damage from oxidative stresses generated by the radicals: the balance between free radicals and antioxidants and the elements controlling the oxidation and reduction reactions in the body.

Excessive amounts of radicals lead to increased levels of oxidative stresses and cell damage. The body naturally has antioxidants that help repair most of the damage, but at these higher levels, the body cannot cope so the damage accumulates undeterred.

The elements controlling the oxidation and reduction reactions in the body determine the balance between free radicals and antioxidants. This, in turn, determines the extent (if any) of cell damage from oxidative stresses generated by excessive amounts of radicals. The body naturally has antioxidants that help repair most of the damage, but at these higher levels, the body cannot cope, so damage accumulates undeterred.

Bioelectricity and Electron Movement

The nervous system controls the physical body by electrical impulses. We know that bioelectricity is traveling throughout our bodies, but what are its pathways, how does it work, and what does it really do?

In the physical world, there are two ways for electrical energy to flow. An electron moves along a conductor when a voltage force acts on it. In addition, electrons move along a semiconductor by jumping from hole to hole. Within the human body, both methods of electron movement occur. The movement of electrons in the semiconductor is similar to the movement of bioelectricity in the body. Free radicals allow bioelectricity to move through the body.

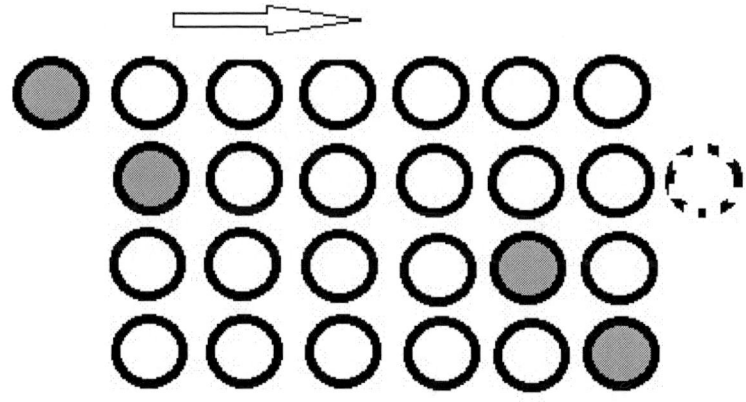

Electron movement is one of the ways for passing energy

In the movement of radicals, the electron from the oxygen atom or the electron in the chain reaction, may act like a domino to pass its energy. The production of radical oxygen, the most common radical in biological systems, occurs mostly within the mitochondria of a cell.

Mitochondria are small membrane-enclosed regions of a cell that produce the chemicals a cell uses for energy. Mitochondria accomplish this task through the electron transport chain mechanism described earlier. Electrons are passed between molecules, producing useful chemical energy with each pass.

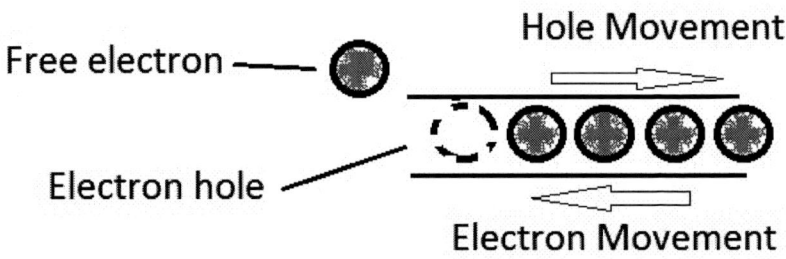

An electron flies out and is then known to be a free electron: what is left is an electron hole which then causes hole movement and electron movement

In the semiconductor, the electron holes are filled by free electrons. If one of the "dominos" is missed or skipped, then the chain reaction will stop.

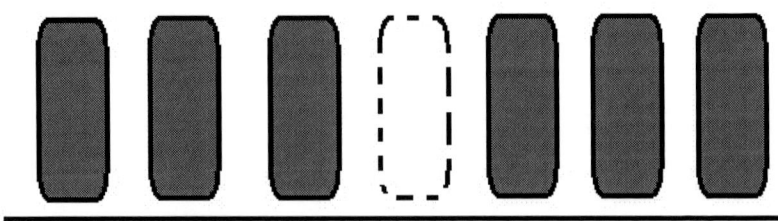

If a domino is skipped or stuck, it will lose its function

The human body follows similar behavior in that the oxygen's proximity to the radical can affect the replacement of the free electron. Radicals are very reactive, but only with those electrons within a few molecules of it. When an organ is in a low-level oxygen condition, there are fewer oxygen atoms to react with the radicals, inhibiting the flow of energy into the organ. This is similar to pushing on the chain of dominos, each one knocks over the next one until it hits on the one area with a missing domino—then the chain reaction stops.

Oxygen in the human body works much like the domino effect. When oxygen levels are low, there are not enough free electrons for the free radicals to fill their electron holes, complete their outer shell with a paired electron, and achieve stability. Low levels of oxygen in an organ can result from poor blood circulation, which may be caused by a faulty nervous system.

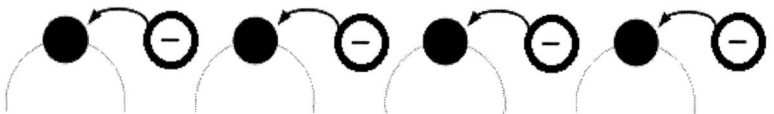

Domino-like Signaling of Free Radicals

Medical research has demonstrated that free radicals and other reactive oxygen species are produced either from normal essential metabolic processes in the body or the body's response to external stimulation such as exposure to X-rays, ozone, cigarette smoking, air pollutants, or industrial chemicals.

We know that radicals are necessary for normal body functions, but too many radicals can be harmful. The body needs to produce an immune response to clean out the excess free radicals.

Getting rid of excess free radicals

Modern medicine has conducted extensive research on free radicals, but how do they treat this problem? The most popular method uses antioxidants, a scavenger that offers free electrons from its hydrogen atoms to pair up with the free electrons in the radicals. By not pairing the radical with oxygen atoms, the oxidative damage is reduced. Other types of antioxidants may inhibit or slow the oxidation process by removing the catalyst involved in the reaction.

Many products claim to clean out free radicals and help with anti-aging. The most common products are BHA and BHT that are added to many foodstuffs to prevent them from rotting or discoloring. Other popular sources are supplements containing vitamins A, C, E, and B.

Medical research has found that though the above antioxidants are beneficial as free radical-fighting scavengers, there are serious side effects to consider. Some research suggests that taking vitamin supplements on a regular basis may interfere with the body's natural production of antioxidants.

People who exercise vigorously use greater amounts of oxygen and produce an increased number of oxidants. Tissue in the body is damaged, the muscles become fatigued, and levels of oxidative stress increase within the body. The body produces more free radicals to use as markers in the process of eliminating the damaged tissue.

In this case, artificially high levels of antioxidants in the body interfere with the function of free radicals and can slow down the body's effort to recover. Other studies show that certain combinations of antioxidant vitamin supplements can have life threatening consequences. In the CARET study, smokers, after taking beta-carotene and vitamin A supplements, showed increased rates of lung cancer.

The human body naturally generates its own antioxidants to keep the number of free radicals in check. However, as discussed earlier, the body can produce an excess amount of radicals and create an imbalance. The best way to clean out the extra radicals is to stop it at those sites within the body where the excess radicals collect.

It is without a doubt that certain vitamins and other antioxidant products can clean out extra free radicals. These methods can replace the oxygen electrons and create balance in the cells, but they may cause a new problem—molecules from the vitamins or scavenger may lose electrons themselves, thus adding a new group of free radicals to the body.

Care must be used when taking vitamin supplements, as an overdose can fill the body with toxins. We know that vitamins A, D, E, and K are difficult for the body to absorb, so when too much is ingested, a skin rash may appear on the upper back, chest, or liver area. The skin condition may be caused by a non-functioning sweat gland or because the liver is toxic from the use of chemical products.

The Tom Tam Healing System believes that the extra free radicals in the body cause degenerative conditions due to a combination of excess free radicals and a condition of oxygen deficiency. Free radicals, present in a normal functional body, depend on the movement of replacement electrons.

When a signal is sent from the brain to the cell and the nearest cell does not carry enough oxygen (or there is not enough oxygen in that area), there are not enough oxygen molecules with free electrons to pair up with to fill the electron hole. If impulse signals continue to come from the brain to this area of low oxygen, the excess free radicals will seek out whatever oxygen or other molecules are nearby to satisfy their need for free electrons. This depletes the oxygen supply in this area even more, but the excess is big enough that the number of free radicals remains high.

In the case of healing, we need to consider both internal and external factors of free radical creation. To balance the intake of oxygen, the first area of attention is the phrenic nerve system. The phrenic nerves radiate from C3, C4, and C5. Its reflex point is on LI17 and we can usually find the blockage of the phrenic nerve on the left hand side. When we lightly press this point, the patient may feel extreme pain.

Because blood carries oxygen to the organs, a circulation problem may cause a condition of oxygen deficiency—this, in turn, may cause free radicals to form. It is impossible to check the efficiency of an individual organ's blood circulation, but we can use the Huatuojaiji points along the spinal column to find the related blockage points.

For example, in people who have a lung problem (including cancer), we can easily find the blockage in the T3 area along the spinal column. If the problem is in the liver, then we find the blockage at T9 on the right-hand side.

The spinal column contains the sympathetic nerve pathways, as well as the spinal artery, so the question arises: is the blockage from the spinal column, the sympathetic nerve, or the spinal artery? We don't know exactly; but we do know that a spinal energy blockage relates to a particular organ.

The superoxide radical (O2) can lead to the production of the very damaging hydroxyl radical (OH). The hydroxyl radical is the most toxic of all the oxygen-based free radicals.

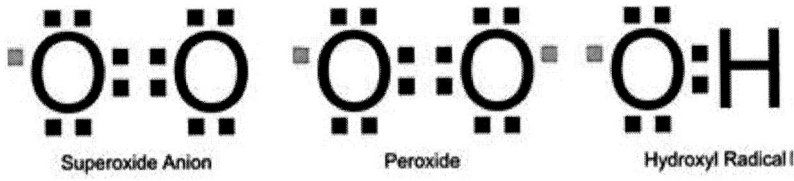

Superoxide Anion   Peroxide   Hydroxyl Radical I

The reaction of oxygen produces heat and metabolism within the body. The warmth produced is from the oxygen reaction. Redness of the skin or palms may be caused by blood cells carrying more oxygen. We cannot use the blood circulation theory alone to explain this feeling of warmth, however, because the free radical function is triggered by the nervous system. If the nervous system is not functioning normally, the amount of oxygen circulating in the body may become irregular.

Free Radicals and Tong Ren Healing

During Tong Ren healing, people most often feel warmth or heat in the body, usually beginning on the face (the face may also turn red). The warm or tingling sensation then runs down to the arm and palms, and may also continue into the chest area. In TCM, this warm or tingling feeling is the body's experience of Chi moving along a meridian. The warmth from Tong Ren healing does not follow the meridian or Chi track from the TCM theory, so this can cause confusion. But if we use free radical theory, it is easier to understand.

In Tong Ren healing, the mind is a powerful and causative force for moving the electron. However, harnessing the power of the mind to affect free radicals requires training and an understanding of how free radical functions in the body.

Each cell within the body reacts about ten thousand times to the free radical movements. In fact, free radicals move in the same direction as the bioelectricity within the body. Bioelectricity is used by the body to transfer metabolic energy. If the flow of bioelectricity is slowed or blocked, the body will not function properly.

Of course, the nervous system controls the movement of the body, its muscles, and sensory organs, but it cannot touch every cell in the body.

The blood vessels or lymph systems, residing near the cells, cannot touch the cells. How, then, can the cells assign the oxygen electron to other cells? We know that the tissue spaces between cells are filled with interstitial fluids (which carry oxygen and hydrogen) and that free radicals signal within this fluid.

According to Tong Ren healing theory, if we can stimulate the body's interstitial fluids, then we can clean the extra oxygen-free electrons that may cause functional imbalance within the body. So how can we stimulate the body to make the fluid active, or balanced?

Western medicine advises people to drink eight glasses of water per day for balance. However, patients with edema or kidney failure cannot drink this much daily—besides, the water we drink daily may not help internal water circulation within the body or organs, so I do not believe this is the answer.

The Kidney's Role in Healing

According to TCM theory, the kidney belongs to the Water element, which maintains and processes the body's fluids. When the kidney's Chi is out of balance, it will cause an internal water problem. The kidney meridian runs from the bottom of the foot, up the leg, abdomen and chest, and then rises to the collarbone. In medical practice, when a patient has a water circulation problem, we can see a distension of the stomach or abdominal area. If swelling occurs in the leg, the puffing is mostly in the Yin meridian located inside the leg.

In TCM theory, the kidney is regarded as the body's most important reservoir of essential energy, forming the basis of life. The kidney system includes the adrenal glands as well as the testicles in men and the ovaries in women—by controlling sexual and reproductive functions, it is the body's prime source of sexual vitality.

According to Western medicine, the kidneys are responsible for filtering waste metabolites from the blood then moving them to the bladder for excretion in urine and, along with the large intestine, for controlling the balance of fluids in the body. In the West, it is a normal procedure to remove a kidney or replace a non-functioning one with a new one when possible.

According to Tong Ren healing, if we stimulate the kidney meridian, it may help the movement of fluids in the body, which can clean out the oxygen-free electrons and balance the free radicals. In TCM, the kidney meridian begins at the bottom of the foot and runs upward to the chest.

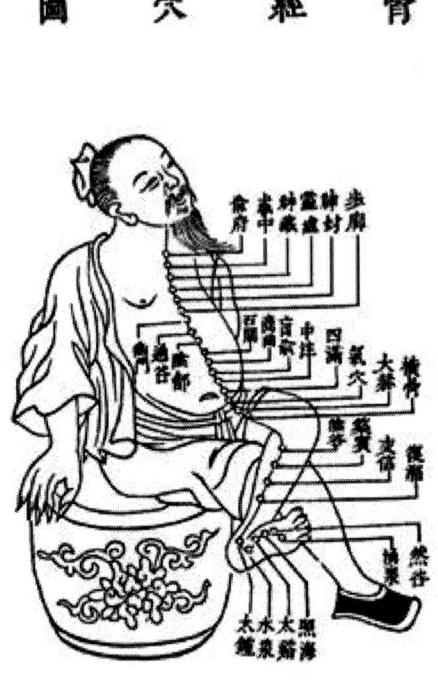

Kidney Meridian

In Tong Ren practice, however, the kidney meridian is opposite, running downward, from top to bottom—we breathe oxygen in through the nose and mouth (at the top of the system) and it flows downward from there.

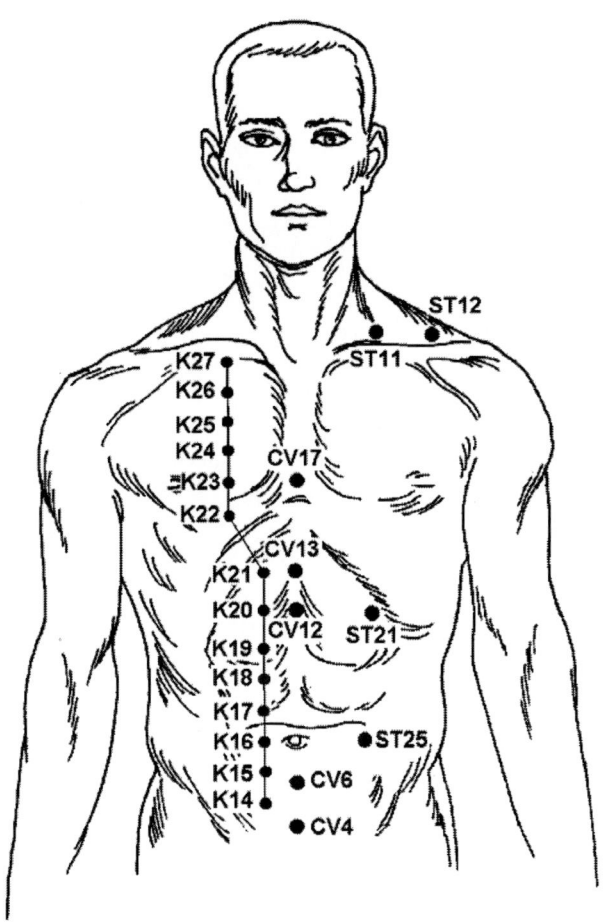

Kidney Meridian Points on the Thorax

The use of Tong Ren healing to open the kidney meridian can heal many diseases because the kidney meridian runs through all the major organs from the abdomen to the chest. If we limit our understanding to modern anatomy, it does not make any sense, but if we consider the electron theory with free radicals and free electrons, it may bring future medicine to a new level.

Telomere and Enzyme

The telomere is the structure at each end of the chromosome, within the cell. It is used much like a helmet is used for protection; it does not play a part in genetic function and does not contain any information itself. The telomere consists of an area of highly repeated DNA combined with protein. Its main function is to help stabilize, and protect the end of the chromosome. When the telomere becomes shorter, the chromosome has less protection from damage.

Normal telomeres allow cells to maintain chromosomes at a normal length. Each time a cell divides, the telomeres get shorter—when the telomeres get too short, the cell can no longer divide and it becomes inactive, senescent, or dies.

Human's cells normally divide only about 50 to 70 times, with telomeres getting progressively shorter until the cells become old or die. In a newborn baby, the telomeres are at their longest, and as their body grows, their cells' telomeres get shorter and shorter.

Studies of telomeres

In 2009, the Nobel Prize in Physiology or Medicine was awarded to a trio of scientists for the discovery of how chromosomes are protected by telomeres and the enzyme telomerase. The recipients were Elizabeth H. Blackburn, Carol W. Greider, and Jack W. Szostak from the United States, but, in fact, the Russian biologist Alexey M. Olovnikov was the first to recognize the problem of telomere shortening and predict the existence of telomerase, in 1973. He also suggested the Telomere Hypothesis of aging and the telomeres' relation to cancer theory.

Today, researchers initiating medical studies regarding the healing of cancer and aging problems are beginning to pay attention to the telomere theory. Of course, right away many companies claim that supplements can fix DNA with the products they sell. Scientific studies on this subject are just beginning, though, and many questions that have been posed cannot yet be answered.

The role of enzymes and telomerase in healing cancer

To help healthy cells last longer or become 'immortal', we need to keep the telomeres long indefinitely. Scientists have discovered that the natural enzyme **telomerase** adds bases to the ends of telomeres which can keep telomeres from wearing down too fast. When cells divide repeatedly, there is not enough telomerase to repair the damage to the telomeres, so they become shorter and the cells age. This enzyme is active in stem cells, germ cells, hair follicles, and 90% of cancer cells, but its expression is low or absent in somatic cells.

Shortened telomeres have been found in many cancers, including pancreatic, bone, prostate, bladder, lung, and kidney cancers. Some doctors wonder whether measuring telomerase may *detect* cancer, and some have tried to stop telomerase activity in cancer cells to *force* those cells to age and die. Yet in the laboratory, researchers found that blocking telomerase also could destroy fertility, wound healing, and the production of blood cells and immune system cells—so work continues.

In order to make healthy cells last longer, attention should be focused on the telomerase, but not the telomere itself. When the telomere wears down too much, the telomerase can repair it. The telomerase can help stem cells and germ cells last longer, but how does it cause cancer cells to grow fast and live longer?

In my understanding, when we go back to the Warburg Effect theory, we may understand how oxygen can cause this to happen. Cancer cells mutate from normal cells or somatic cells. When the normal cells lack the necessary oxygen, they must be in the fermentation process in order survive.

Somatic cells have low amounts, or even an absence of, telomerase—yet 90% of cancerous cells have telomerase in a greater, or at least substantial, quantity. In fact, cancer cells have mutated from normal cells; the difference between the two is their oxygen level.

In the Warburg Effect theory, we know that when normal cells have low or no oxygen for a period of 48 hours, they can become cancerous. If so, then we can easily understand that the yeast which is an enzyme can mutate quickly when in a low oxygen state. This theory is exhibited in the same way that mushrooms grow: if there is plenty of sunshine and oxygen, the mushroom cannot grow well.

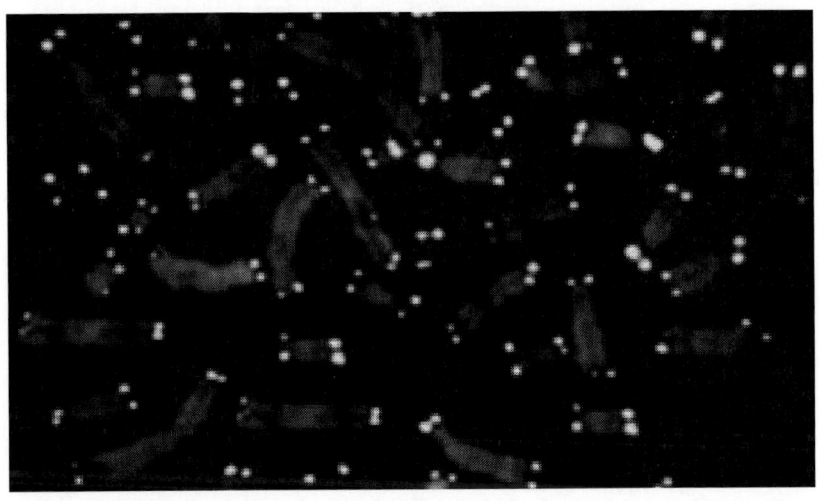

Telomeres cap and protect the ends of chromosomes

Enzymes are one of the most interesting and important substances found in nature. Enzymes are not living things; they are just like minerals, which are inanimate. But unlike minerals, they are created by living cells. They are natural proteins that stimulate and accelerate many biological reactions in the body.

In the human body, there are two types of enzyme. One helps join specific molecules together to form new molecules; the other helps break specific molecules apart into separate molecules. Enzymes play many important roles outside the cells as well. When the cells have telomerase, it does not mean that a chemical reaction will take place.

Chemical alteration of a substance within the body is by the action of enzymes, yet many enzymes will *not* work without the presence of an *additional, non-protein* substance called a **cofactor**. If the cofactor is organic, it is called a **coenzyme**. Coenzymes are relatively small molecules compared to the protein part of the enzyme. Many coenzymes are derived from vitamins, and for this reason, many alternative cancer healing theories are based on the use of enzymes and vitamins.

Enzyme therapy for healing cancer involves taking enzyme supplements. These supplements often consist of combinations of several enzymes and come in pill, capsule, or powder form, yet no established safe or effective dosage has been determined. Human cells naturally produce about 10,000 different enzymes which are essential in normal metabolism, so using supplement therapy to heal cancer is like playing a lottery—you may choose the right ones and win, but what is the *probability* of doing that? Using enzyme supplements to heal cancer is similar to using vitamins—before the patient uses this type of treatment, they should consider this: what is the probability of healing, or what is the healing rate?

Lately, cancer healing studies have many new theories. Many clinical trials test a form of Targeted Cancer Therapy, which is killing cancer cells, or interfering with the growth of the cancer cells, but doing nothing to the healthy cells. It is a good idea and theory, but does it really work or is it just a dream? Ten years ago, my book *Tong Ren for Cancer* addressed this type of healing. Many cancer patients and doctors have put great hope in this healing, yet after many years and countless case studies, this type of healing is still in a clinical trial.

In the laboratory, the Targeted Cancer Therapies, sometimes called *molecularly targeted drugs*, or molecularly targeted therapy, works well with mice, but in clinical practice for human cancer patients there is a significant difference in the results. It is easy to understand why: the mice received a man-made cancer, but humans get cancer from their body being out of balance naturally. In the lab, cancer in mice can be healed even without any treatment.

Some targeted therapies (drugs called signal transduction inhibitors) block specific enzymes, or telomerase and growth factor receptors, involved in cancer cell proliferation. The use of drugs to repair enzymes is not an easy job, because the human body has so many different enzymes. An easy and effective method is to improve the oxygen condition of the cells.

If we limit the method for targeting cancer cells with a drug, it may work temporarily, but if the body's enzymes grow faster than the drug's killing rate, then new cell growth is still mutating in the wrong way. It's just like someone's basement that has too much mold or allergy-causing bacteria; the way to clean out the mold is to open the window and let in more air flow and sunshine, not to use chemical sprays to cover up the problem. Using the Telomerase inhibitor as cancer therapy is a wonderful idea, but it has a long way to go.

Telomere and telomerase are involved in the mutation process of cells and cancer is a direct result of this process. The cell mutation process has many contributing factors, including: blood circulation, oxygen, growth hormone, bioelectricity, free radical, metabolism, and the immune system. The confusing or complex piece of this process is found in the difference between stem cells and germ cells, compared with other cells in the body—they need telomerase to keep the telomere long, and other normal cells do not.

In the human body, each cell has its own function and genetic makeup. We cannot change the cells' genes nor force them to grow under control. Telomeres in mice cannot cause their normal cells to become cancerous cells. This has been proven, and speaks to the discussion that scientists currently have around the fear of creating cancer cells. In the laboratory, telomeres will not react in a way that causes cells to become cancerous. Only the body's normal cells, when oxygen and biochemical changes occur, can turn cancerous.

The focus of medical studies of telomeres is on the subject of age and cancer. However, scientists discovered that telomeres can cause many other diseases, such as heart problems, diabetes, weight problems, Alzheimer's disease, hypertension, elderly onset rheumatoid arthritis (EORA), arrhythmia, and cerebrovascular accident. Of course, as scientific studies continue developing, they will find more diseases which may be caused from the telomere theory.

Points for telomeres stimulation

In my theory, the belief is that any telomere growth is related to growth hormone. Growth hormone is controlled from the hypothalamus and pituitary gland, located in the brain. The associated energy points to use are GV22 and GV23. To have a wider healing effect in this area, we also use BL6.

Combined with these points, we should make use of the kidney meridian when we implement Tong Ren healing. In administering an acupuncture treatment, we don't need to use the whole kidney meridian, use only K16 and LV3 which stimulate free radical function in the body. When we open the blockage to balance the telomere and telomerase, we must open the blockage on the phrenic nerve first, because the phrenic nerve's function can balance the oxygen level in the body. If the oxygen doesn't function well in the body, it may affect the function of telomerase.

When working to heal cancer patients, use the points in the frontal lobe as the last step for treatment. Also, stimulation of BL6, GV22, GV23, LV3 and the kidney meridian can be used as the last step in Tong Ren healing, or in the case of a Chi Gong practice or Chi Gong healing it can be used along with the closing movement.

The kidney meridian points can lead the Chi to the toes which, in effect, leads the Chi to the ground. Also, we can picture leading the extra free radicals to the ground and out of the body. In any case, opening the kidney meridian points can smooth and slow down energy movement, which brings the body back to a normal energy circulation state.

Traditional Chinese Medicine believes that the mind and body cannot be separated in the healing practice. Also, the scientific studies prove that severe and chronic emotional stress may cause the telomeres to become shorter.

For the purpose of healing, and for a long life, we should keep a relaxed mind—this will affect the circulation and function of the brain which will then have a physiological effect on the body. This can also explain the studies which support Tai Chi, Qi Gong, and meditation playing an important role in creating this effect on the mind and body.

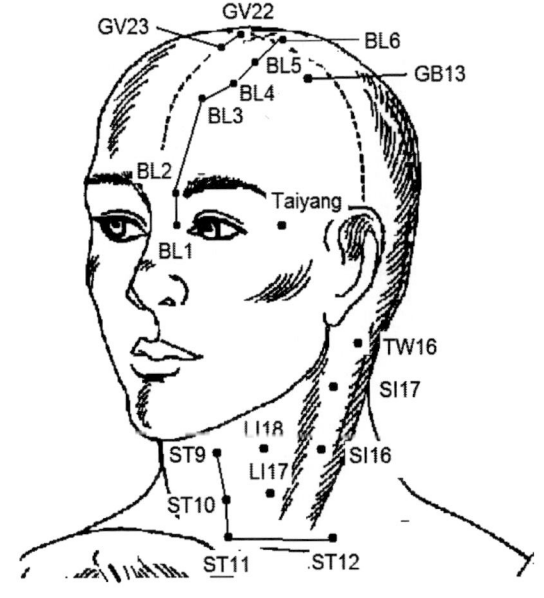

The brain's role in healing

The brain controls two important functions—one is the psychological function and other is the physical. The brain makes up only 2% of the total mass of the human body, but it needs 20% of the body's blood circulation.

The brain's blood circulation is limited by the size of the two arteries which support the brain: the common carotid and vertebral arteries. It also is dependent on the blood flow amount and blood pressure.

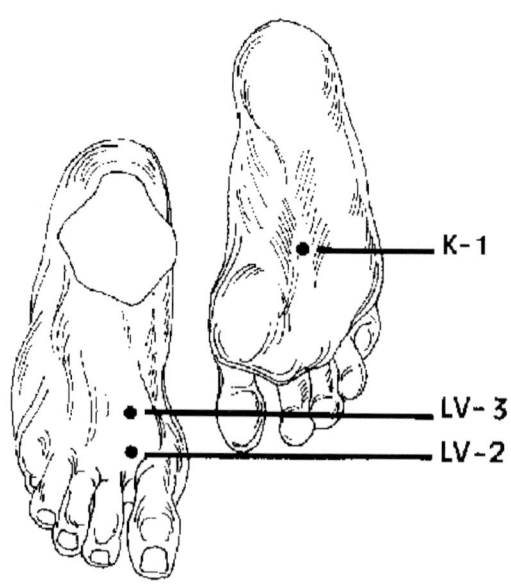

K1 and LV3

Yet, these two arteries are not limited only by their physiological function; they can also be limited by any constriction in the body. If blood circulation runs more effectively to the psychological centers in the brain, then the physical part of the brain will receive less.

When people experience high stress then the brain may need more blood circulation to the psychological part of the brain, but this can cause less circulation to the physical control centers in the brain.

When we are focusing on healing cancer patients, we need to pay attention to calming down the mind which can help divert the focus of blood circulation more to the physical control center of the brain. For this healing, we can use the GB13, BL1, BL2 and BL3 points in the frontal lobe area.

This aspect of the treatment has valuable functional implications on the body. When the mind is calm, the physical body can heal.

Neocortex and Gallbladder Meridian

All studies relating to causes of cancer focus on DNA and biochemical factors. Rarely can one find a study that pays attention to the *bioelectrical* factors involved. In my studies, I focus on the nervous system—this is the network of bioelectricity in the body, or in other words the *biosignal pathway*.

The reason I pay attention to bioelectricity is very simple. Scientifically speaking, the body has two routes to pass the biosignal: biochemical and bioelectric. If we invest in biochemical studies and get no positive feedback, should we not look to find an alternate method? Scientific research is to search the unknown world, without being limited by any preconceived notions.

In my understanding of cancer treatment there is a blockage on the nerve. This blockage may interfere with the absorption of oxygen and the flow of bioelectricity to the organ. My theory is a belief that the oxygen intake is from the phrenic nerve, and the organ's bioelectricity current is from the autonomic nerve's function.

In order for any cell to become cancerous, it must have these two factors: oxygen deficiency and low voltage, or current, of bioelectricity.

The human body is formed by millions of individual cells, each functioning like a battery, storing energy. This energy's function is controlled by the biosignal from the brain, which can be measured and monitored using specialized equipment. The term *biosignal* is often used to mean bioelectrical signal. In fact, the biosignal refers to both electrical and non-electrical signals. In medical studies for healing cancer, most medical experts and laboratories favor *non*-electrical signals such as chemical, mechanical, acoustic, and optical signals.

Electrical biosignals are usually understood to be electric currents produced by the sum of electrical potential differences across a specialized tissue, organ, or cell system such as the nervous system. To understand the function of bioelectrical signal in the body, we must first understand Ohm's law. According to Ohm's law, **I =V/R**. I is the electric current or the strength of energy flowing in the body. If the voltage potential (V) does not change, then the R (resistance) can change the electric current's flow (I). The body's nerve is the cable which acts as the passageway for the current conductor. When the nerve has a high resistance, the organ's electric current will be lowered.

The brain is formed by billions of neurons. It is the command center and main information center of the entire body. When the brain sends out an abnormal signal, the body's function will also be abnormal. If the brain gets damaged (such as by a stroke), it may cause the body's function to lose control. When the motor cortex gets damaged, the body's movement may also lose its function or have abnormal movement.

When the Broca's area gets damaged, the patient may lose speech function. In medical studies, cell growth not only depends on growth of hormones, it also relies on the bioelectricity of the brain. The growth hormone and biosignal are both from the brain's functions—if this function is abnormal, then the cell growth may be abnormal as well.

A computer and the human brain function in similar ways. When a computer has a virus, the computer's programs can change their function for the worst. The human brain can have the same thing happen, with the wrong signal playing the role of a virus and causing cells to grow abnormally. The question is: where in the brain is this abnormal function that causes the cells to become cancerous?

This is not an easy question to answer, and so far no one in the medical field has been interested in finding out. Of course, I have the interest although do not have the power and ability to run a medical research lab. The only thing I can do is build up the theory first, then let the next generation finish my theory—my hope is that they will have the interest as well as the power.

We must understand the brain's function in order to discover what part of the brain causes the wrong biosignal to create a cancer. One common phenomenon within the animal world is that animals with a neocortex may develop cancer—an animal without a neocortex simply does not develop cancer. No one to date has paid attention to this relationship between the neocortex and the cause of cancer. My theory still has not been proved by the scientific world; however it is a logical hypothesis for cancer healing.

So What is the Neocortex?

The neocortex is a part of the mammalian brain that stems from the cerebral cortex. The neocortex is Latin for "new rind or "new bark", also called the neopallium or the isocortex. The neocortex is the outer layer of the cerebral hemispheres, and is made up of six layers, labeled I to VI. In the human brain, 90% of the cerebral cortex is neocortex and it is more developed in mammals than non-mammals. The human neocortex is involved in higher level functions which other mammals do not possess, such as sensory perception, generation of motor commands, spatial reasoning, conscious thought, and language.

The neocortex is divided into frontal, parietal, occipital, and temporal lobes, each of which performs a different function. How can we know which lobe may relate to cell growth?

We know that growth hormone is produced from the pituitary gland which is an endocrine gland connected to the hypothalamus. Hormonal function in the body cannot be triggered until it receives the impulse of biosignal from the brain.

Question: what part of the brain creates the biosignal from the nervous system to trigger the hormone? Western medicine developed a method for replacing the hormone for healing, but not the biosignal from the nerve system to trigger the hormone. In fact, in a medical study it was found that psychological activity and physical activity can cause biochemical change as well as brainwave change.

To understand more about the neocortex, we should first understand the central sulcus. The central sulcus is a prominent landmark of the brain, separating the parietal lobe from the frontal lobe, and the primary motor cortex from the primary somatosensory cortex. It is a fold in the cerebral cortex of a vertebrate brain.

The central sulcus is also called the central fissure. It was originally called the fissure of Rolando or the Rolandic fissure, after the Italian anatomist Luigi Rolando who devoted his life to the study of brain anatomy.

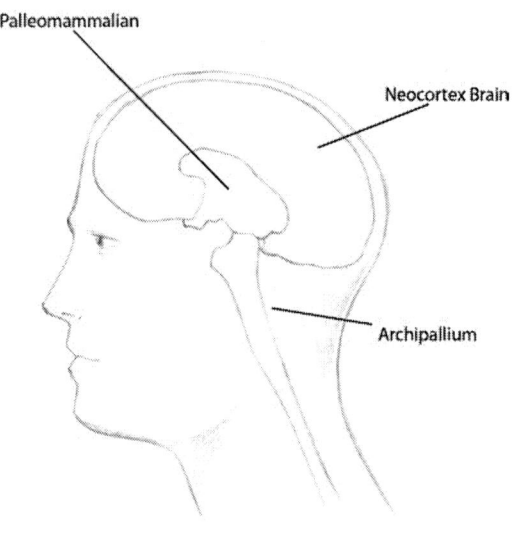

Neocortex brain

Located in the central sulcus' frontal lobe is the motor cortex, and in its parietal lobe is the sensory cortex. All of the body's voluntary movements are controlled by the brain. The motor cortex is heavily involved in controlling these voluntary movements. The motor cortex and sensory cortex work together and cannot be separated. In practice, we should consider stimulating both to maximize each of their functions.

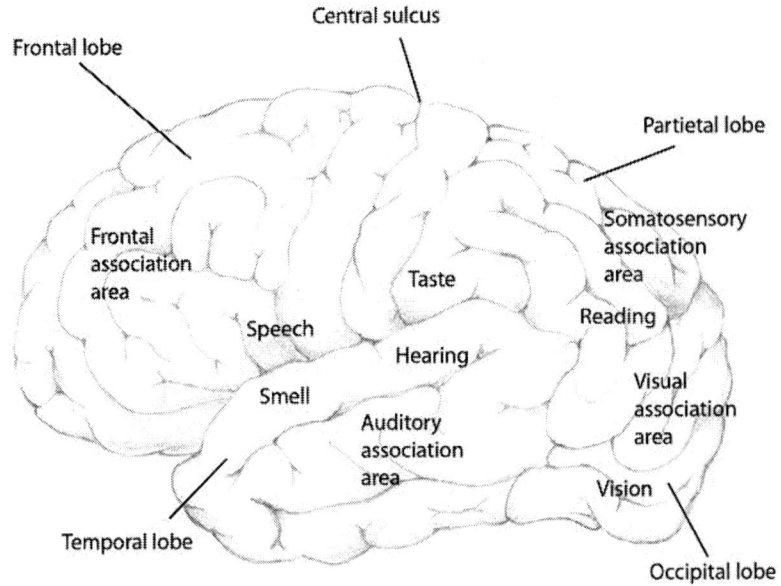

The Central Sulcus

In 1870, a German anatomist, anthropologist Gustav Fritsch together with a neurologist and neuropsychiatrist, Eduard Hitzig, electrically stimulated various parts of a dog's motor cortex. They observed that depending on what part of the cortex they stimulated, a different part of the body contracted. Then, they found that if they destroyed this same small area of the cortex, the corresponding part of the body became paralyzed.

The same reaction occurs in the human body— when the motor cortex is injured (such as by a stroke), then the various parts of the body may stop their normal function or even completely lose function. Also, the same can happen in the sensory cortex as in the motor cortex. When the sensory cortex in the parietal lobe gets damaged, it may cause a sensory problem in various parts of the body.

In medical study, when scientists stimulated the sensory or motor cortexes with a weak electrical current, they found that the stimulation often produced tingling or movement in part of the body. Following the body's reaction from the stimulation, scientists can draw a map as to which parts of the brain control various parts of the body. The mapping is called the Homunculus, which in Latin means "little man." The first homunculus diagram was drawn by Wilder Penfield in the 1940s.

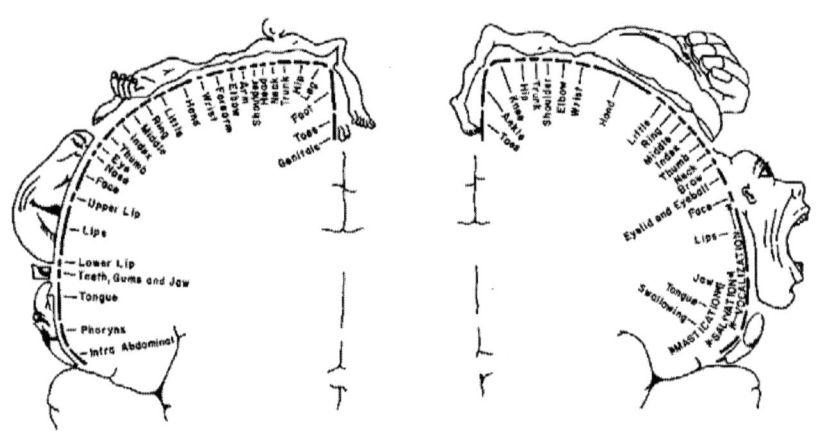

Sensory cortex and motor cortex of Homunculus

A weakened electrical current to the motor cortex or sensory cortex can cause different parts of the body to have a reaction. On the other hand, *stimulation* of the motor or sensory cortex can *strengthen* the current, which can result in healing. In Western medicine, surgery and electrical stimulation of the motor cortex are used for chronic neuropathic pain control.

Currently, scientists also use a strong magnetic field to stimulate areas of the brain for healing. In China, scalp acupuncture is used, in which needles are used to stimulate the scalp for healing. Scalp acupuncture is becoming increasingly popular in the East. It doesn't matter if it is Western or Eastern medicine, each has their own technique and theory to stimulate the scalp for healing purposes. Scalp acupuncture theory is based on the Brodmann areas, which are regions of the cerebral cortex based on its cytoarchitecture, or structure and organization of cells. This method of healing was developed in 1958 by a medical doctor in China.

The following diagram represents a slice of the cortex near the fissure of Rolando. This is the motor cortex of the homunculus. This runs from the top of the head down toward the ear. There has not been any correlation between the motor cortex and the function of the internal organs found. In TCM the internal organs are called Zang-Fu. Scalp acupuncture is very limited because the motor and sensory cortexes don't include the Zang-Fu organ. Mostly the scalp acupuncture is often used to treat cerebral diseases. In the late practice of scalp acupuncture, many systems combined the meridian theory in order to treat the Zang-Fu organ diseases. Yet, its healing rate results are still low for healing the Zang-Fu organ problem.

If we believe that the magnetic field, electrical current, and acupuncture can stimulate the scalp for healing, then we can use these with Tong Ren and Chi Gong to stimulate the scalp for healing as well. While the Western method and theory of stimulating the scalp for healing is accepted by science, Chinese scalp acupuncture continues to be denied by Western skeptics—but this rejection cannot stop the practice and development of scalp acupuncture.

In Western medical practice, evidence is always required—proved from scientific studies. Yet, in Eastern medical practice, little attention is paid to evidence and science, more to the healing result. In the Tom Tam Healing System, though nothing has been proven through medical studies, we do have the results of healed patients and their smiles. No need to argue, we believe the medical evidence already may be controlled by the drug companies, and medical study is not in our range of ability.

In the medical studies, scientists found that when they stimulate the motor cortex, the associated internal organ has the reaction and movement as well. In animal experiments, when electrical stimulation of the neocortex is used, beside the physical movement, it can also cause other reactions that lead to changes in visceral activity.

When stimulating the interior precentral gyrus (located in the motor cortex area) a movement and reaction in the rectum and bladder may occur. Stimulating the exterior precentral gyrus may cause a variation in breathing and movement in the vessels. Stimulating the bottom part of exterior precentral gyrus' may cause gastrointestinal movement and a change in saliva secretion. The same reactions were found through animal studies and in humans.

In Chinese scalp acupuncture, the motor cortex and sensory cortex from the homunculus are used for healing. However, this scalp healing is limited to the external movement from the nervous system as shown in the diagram.

According to these diagrams, we cannot explain why the internal organs can be affected. In the diagram from the motor cortex, we can find out that # 15 (neck) to # 22 (swallowing) is the range that covers the cranial nerves' function. In the diagram from #19 (lips) to #20 (jaw) there is a big gap and has no note for any organ. In other words, according to medical explanations, speech and movement of the jaw require much more space in the brain in order to accomplish these movements.

My theory is different. If this extended area of the brain is the function area for the cranial nerves, then something is missing, primarily dealing with the vagus nerve. In the cranial nerve system, #10 is the vagus nerve which controls the function of many internal organs. If the vagus nerve is connected to the motor cortex, then we can explain why stimulation to the motor cortex can cause a reaction in the internal organs.

Between the gap from #19 to #20 in the motor cortex is the acupuncture point GB8. In my practice, when I use the acupuncture needle to stimulate GB8, most of the patients can feel the warmth or Chi move down as the path or track of the vagus nerve from the opposite side of the body. This energy movement also can cause organ movement from the vagus nerve and result in healing.

What needs to be considered is that no one knows for sure that the GB8 area is associated with the vagus nerve, because we need a scientist who can prove it. The other possibility for the GB8 area is the connection of the neck function. In my theory, LI18 is the vagus nerve location and LI17 is the phrenic nerve location—and both are on the neck. The stimulation of GB8 for the motor cortex area can affect the movement or create a reaction in the jaw and lips. If so, it can be easy to understand why stimulation of GB8 can cause the Chi or energy going down to the chest, stomach, and abdomen, which are the vagus and phrenic nerve pathways.

In ancient Chinese acupuncture, it was believed that GB8 is an intersection point of the Gallbladder and Bladder meridians. This point is indicated for cold and phlegm in the diaphragm and stomach, injury by alcohol, and agitation and fullness with ceaseless vomiting.

All of these conditions are related to the vagus and phrenic nerves. Also, the bottom part of the sensory cortex is for the intra-abdominal, the lower part of the vagus nerve, and for function of the phrenic nerve as well. The intra-abdominal area in TCM is called the lower Dantian where the Chi is stored.

In my healing theory, a nerve acts as a cable which is a pathway of bioelectricity to each organ. To open the blockage of the nerve is to release its resistance, which affects the bioelectricity current by raising it. When stimulated, the scalp, along with the neocortex, may increase the voltage of the bioelectricity.

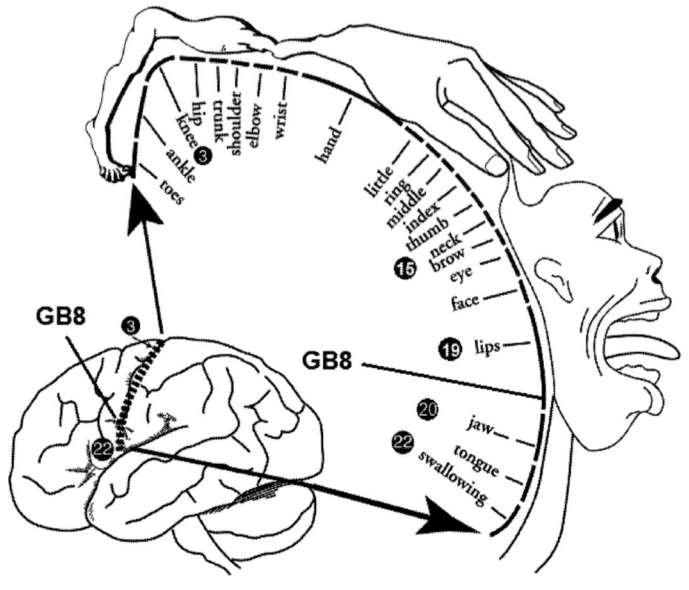

The Motor Cortex of Homunculus and GB8

In clinical practice for healing cancer, when we stimulate GB8 on the side opposite that of the tumor, then the patient who has breast cancer can feel the warmth or Chi movement around the shoulder and breast area. If the patient has pain or feels uncomfortable, they may feel the syndrome change and feel better. If the breast cancer patient has related shoulder problems, she may feel the pain lessen or disappear, and the range of shoulder movement should increase also.

When we heal the cancer case, GB8 is only a part of the choice to raise the bioelectricity's voltage; the other consideration, more importantly, is to open the blockage on the nerve system, which can lower the resistance to allow more bio-current flow. We don't know if stimulating GB8 directly affects the vagus and phrenic nerves, or the neck area, but this is not important—the importance lies with the energy passing through this area which results in healing.

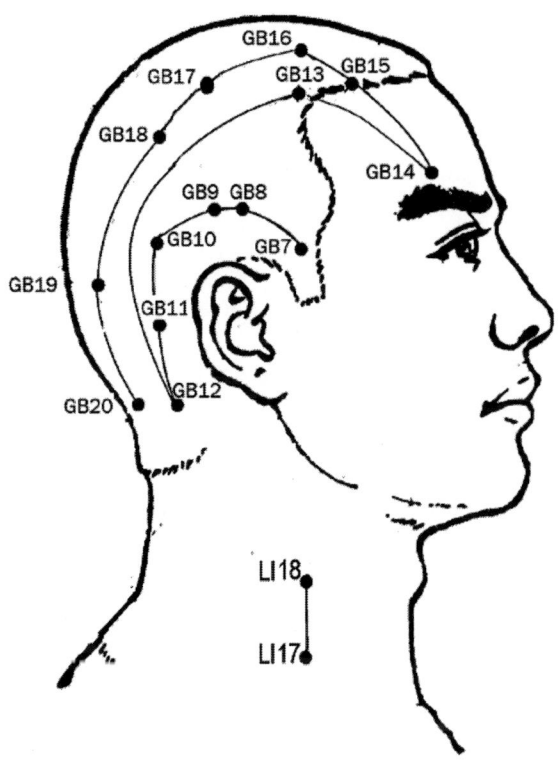

Gallbladder Meridian Points on the Scalp

In addition to GB8, there are other points to consider along the gallbladder meridian on the scalp. For healing cancer or other internal problems, we can use GB7, GB8, and GB9 together to strengthen the healing benefit. If a patient has a leg and hand problem at the same time, we can add GB17 and GB18. Also, BL7 and BL8 are other points that relate to the motor cortex and sensory cortex. Many cancer patients need emotional support and help with staying calm. We can then use GB13, GB14, GB15, and GB16 for relaxation.

The Central Nervous System is made up of the spinal cord and brain. The spinal cord conducts sensory information from the peripheral nervous system with both somatic and autonomic nerves. It also passes motor information from the brain to the various effectors. So when we stimulate the brain, the spinal cord can receive the biosignal and cause a reaction. Conversely, when we stimulate the somatic and autonomic nerves, this may cause activity in the brain. When we are treating cancer, GB8 doesn't work alone; it must be used with other points. In our healing practice, we need to consider various aspects of the nervous system such as the autonomic and cranial nerves.

The gallbladder meridian on the head follows a strange track. Many TCM experts are confused as to why this track runs so crooked. In fact, it is easy to remember how this strange track twists and turns.

We know the neocortex is the outer layer of the cerebral hemispheres which is made up of six layers, labeled from I to VI. A diagram of the meridian system separates the six layers in the skull for us.

We can follow the first layer along the triple warmer meridian around the outer edge of the ear. The second layer is followed by the gallbladder meridian from GB7 to GB12. The third layer is from GB12 to GB14. The forth layer is from GB14 to GB20. The fifth layer goes from the bladder meridian points BL4 to BL9. The last one, the sixth layer, is on the top of scalp, along the governing vessel meridian. This way of division according to the meridians on the scalp is not necessarily anatomically correct, but it is an easy way to remember their locations.

Discovering the Cause of Cancer

Many theories attempt to explain the reason why cancer forms in the body, and each healing system has its own explanation. Some believe that diet or ingested chemicals may cause it. Some believe that our environment contributes to the problem, and others believe that emotions are a causal factor. Traditional Chinese Medicine believes that the human body's internal Chi becomes out of balance, or that "external devil chi" may be the culprit.

Some medical doctors believe genetic factors can predispose a person to cancer, although medical studies to date have failed to conclusively prove this theory. Some studies find that CT scans, X-rays, radiation, chemotherapy, and any number of drugs can cause cancer. In theory, when we find the cause of disease, we can eradicate the disease, but so far, the medical and scientific communities know only some of the factors that may relate to the cause of cancer.

Though the medical field devotes much money, time, and attention to fighting and preventing cancer, the cancer rate has not been lowered. On the contrary, results of current medical studies indicate that the cancer rate continues to rise each year and, today, one out of four Americans is diagnosed with cancer during their lifetime. Logically, we are taught to believe that supporting medical studies will result in a lower rate of cancer, however, experts continue to study their concepts for cancer prevention and still find the cancer rate rising.

In the 1920's, a German doctor discovered that the primary cause of cancer was *the replacement of the respiration of oxygen in normal body cells by a fermentation of sugar.* In 1931, Dr. Otto H. Warburg was awarded the Nobel Prize for research on the respiration of cells by a group of enzymes involved in aerobic (with oxygen) respiration of healthy cells.

Dr. Otto H. Warburg believed that, "Cancer, above all other diseases, has countless secondary causes. But, even for cancer, there is only one *prime* cause. Summarized in a few words, the prime cause of cancer is the replacement of the respiration of oxygen in normal body cells by a fermentation of sugar."

In other words, cancer is not caused by a virus, nor is it a basic cell problem—it is caused by a *lack of oxygen* in cells. Why would cells lack oxygen? Many things can cause low oxygen levels: oxygen intake may be low for some reason, or a circulation problem may interfere with the transportation of oxygen to the body's cells.

Dr. Warburg states that, "All normal cells have an absolute requirement for oxygen, but cancer cells can live without oxygen—a rule without exception...Deprive a cell of 35% of its oxygen for 48 hours and it may become cancerous." He discovered that cancer cells are anaerobic—they do not breathe oxygen and cannot survive in the presence of high levels of oxygen.

In Dr. Warburg's work, *"The Metabolism of Tumors,"* he demonstrated that all forms of cancer are characterized by two basic conditions: acidosis and anaerobic condition (lack of oxygen). They are two sides of the same coin—where you have one, you have the other.

How cancer cells can live without oxygen is a good question. We understand that any normal cell which loses its supply of oxygen must find another source of energy if it is to survive. The cell has two resources from which to obtain its energy: oxygen and the fermentation of sugar. It is similar to a hybrid car, in which the battery supplies the energy, but when the battery is low, gasoline supplies its energy instead.

Dr. Warburg discovered that, "Cancer cells are dormant in a pH environment slightly above 7.4. In a pH 8.5+ environment, cancer cells die while healthy cells thrive." Some healing methods use the pH and acid theory to attempt to understand cancer cell growth. Some patients are advised to eat an alkaline diet to create an alkaline condition in the body. Yet these methods fail to correct an oxygen deficiency. They can correct pH, but they do not correct the primary cause of cancer: the deprivation of oxygen.

Some experts believe that carbon monoxide, which reduces the oxygen-carrying capacity of blood, may be a cause of cancer. Fluoride interferes with oxygen uptake and is also viewed as a culprit. Alcohol and drugs rob the body of oxygen because the body must oxidize these substances during the process of their removal. Indeed, many external factors can affect cancer risk, but they are *not* the main cause.

A malfunction of the phrenic nerve is the major factor causing oxygen intake to be out of balance. Traditional Chinese Medicine does not recognize oxygen, but it recognizes that air is considered life force. Therefore, TCM understands air as a part of the formation of Chi, or energy.

In Chinese writing, Chi and air are the same character. When any human being is without air, the Chi is gone. When the air content decreases in the body, the Chi is low. Chi is stored in a point called the Dantian.

There are many questions about the causes of cancer and I cannot give a definitive answer; we need scientists to study and find the answer. So far, all of the studies focus on chemicals for commercial purpose or scientific research, but no one is interested in such things as the nerve systems, the diaphragm, or bioelectricity in relation to cancer healing. My hope is that someday someone will bravely change this.

I believe that cancer is caused from the phrenic nerve and autonomic nerves—and someday we are going to prove it.

Warburg's Findings Gain Attention

More scientists are showing interest in the Warburg effect. In Canada, the University of Alberta is testing a drug called dichloroacetate which suppresses the Warburg effect and reactivates mitochondria. The result shows why mitochondrial suppression is so important to tumors: when mitochondria are unsuppressed, the tumor they're in stops growing.

And at Harvard Medical School, Dr. Fantin and Dr. Leder are working with RNA interference to modify glycolysis in the tumors of specially bred laboratory mice. RNA interference is the subject of eager investigation among pharmaceutical companies, but so far it has yet to yield a drug approved by regulators.

In June 1966, Dr. Warburg wrote *The Prime Cause and Prevention of Cancer*, stating, "To prevent cancer it is therefore proposed first to keep the speed of the blood stream so high that the venous blood still contains sufficient oxygen; second, to keep high the concentration of hemoglobin in the blood; third, to add always to the food, even of healthy people, the active groups of the respiratory enzymes (the 4 nutrients); and to increase the doses of these groups, if a precancerous state has already developed. If at the same time exogenous carcinogens are excluded rigorously, then much of the endogenous cancer may be prevented today."

People mainly want to kill cancer cells by any available method or philosophy. The methods used to kill already-present cancer cells are simple, but to prevent the growth of *new* cancer cells is difficult, if not impossible. Interference to stop glycol can kill cancer cells, however, if the patient's condition does not improve, new normal cells will continue to mutate into cancerous ones.

In fact, when scientists use a killing method for healing cancer, it may worsen oxygen intake. On the other hand, if normal cells are provided with sufficient oxygen, they will not become cancerous.

Trying to Unlock the Cause of Cancer

Western medicine has advanced systems and techniques for disease research and healing. In external-factor cancer studies, the West commissions huge financial investments and top research scientists in an attempt to find causes of cancer from the environment: air and water pollution, x-rays, and chemicals. Many factors can affect cancer growth in our bodies, but the environmental ones are only secondary—we have yet to find the primary cause.

Cancer is not a virus and it is not a germ; I contend that it is simply a cell with a low voltage of bioelectricity and lack of oxygen. Cancer cells are inactive (meaning that they do not carry enough bioelectricity to function normally) and they are undernourished; therefore, they mutate quickly. Killing cancer cells is an easy job, but stopping normal cells from mutating into cancer cells is nearly impossible.

Most cancer research consists of internal-factor studies focused on DNA. The latest theory believes that cancer is the result of accumulated mutations to a cell's DNA. It was first proposed by Carl O. Nordling in 1953 and later formulated in 1971 by Alfred George Knudson, Jr., M.D., Ph.D., a geneticist specializing in cancer genetics. Knudson's work led indirectly to the identification of cancer-related genes which explains the effects of mutation on carcinogenesis (the development of cancer).

Does DNA Play a Role?

Before we talk about DNA, first we must know what DNA is. DNA, or deoxyribonucleic acid, is the nucleic acid that contains the genetic instructions used in the development and functioning of all known living organisms. Nearly every cell in a person's body has the same DNA. Chemically, DNA consists of two long polymers of simple units called nucleotides with backbones made of sugars and phosphate groups.

In current Western medical studies, most attention focuses on DNA research as doctors and scientists try to discover the secret of the cancer cell. Realize, however, that DNA studies are limited to understanding the *structure of chemicals inside* the cell, and do *not* include any consideration of the *electricity* within the cell.

According to medical studies, many experts focus their studies on cells in an attempt to discover how cancer cells and tumors are formed, and to understand the intricacies of how DNA and RNA cells change. Scientists are excited that their high technological expertise may provide answers for this postulate. Millions of dollars are invested and countless experts work hard to find the answers.

When cancer is discussed, many people automatically assume there is a tumor. Indeed, cancer often does present itself in the form of a tumor or as a cellular problem, but not always. For example, in leukemia (a cancer of the blood or bone marrow), the body is flooded with immature blood cells or the blood cells mutate.

Discoveries about DNA provide valuable clues that help police solve crimes, but, unfortunately, they can never help heal cancer. DNA research cannot help us heal cancer or understand cell mutation because DNA research is focused on only one part of the cell, not the complete story behind the disease.

Native American indigenous science believes that all life began from lightning and thunder. Of course, modern science laughs at this philosophy. I believe that the first organic cell was produced from an inorganic chemical "soup" heated in a watery environment and then energized (transformed) by electrical discharge. So, when research is conducted on cells or DNA or genes, the cell's electrical charge should not be eliminated from the experimental protocol.

During cell research, cells are isolated from the body in an artificial medium in the lab—away from the natural, organic bioelectricity from the body—while cells in the body are always enmeshed in bioelectric energy. The result is that the cells in the lab and the cells in the body are being tested under completely different conditions. We can only understand a problem like cancer from the context of the entire organism, the whole body including it bioelectricity.

If a DNA test is performed outside the body, its results should not be used in medical practice because the cells have been removed from their natural setting: the human body with its ever-present bioelectricity. Consider this: a cell in a laboratory is like meat in a refrigerator; it is completely different than the meat which is growing on a living animal's body. How can the results from one be used to heal the other? The answer is simple: they can't.

The synergy between the biochemistry and bioelectricity within the cell of a living body is entirely different from the "Petri dish" of the refrigerator. Studies on mice are not transferable to human subjects because the cancer in the mice has been caused artificially (chemically), not by natural conditions. In double-blind experiments in a laboratory, tumors can spontaneously disappear from "control" subject mice, (meaning, those who received no treatment whatsoever), leaving the scientists wondering, "how did it disappear?"

In Tong Ren theory, the answer is because the cancer was man-made, rather than caused by a blockage. The mouse's nerve function was still normal, so the nervous and endocrine systems still had the ability to collect abnormal DNA genes and pump out healthy cells via growth hormones, thus allowing auto-repair.

It has been found that carcinogenesis depends both on the activation of proto-oncogenes (genes that stimulate cell proliferation) and the deactivation of tumor suppressor genes (genes that keep proliferation in check).

Can the Somatic Nervous System Cause Cancer?

Because all cells throughout the body are controlled by nervous system impulses, we should ask whether the somatic (motor) nervous system could possibly be a cancer-causing factor. I believe it is.

The motor nervous system (motor pathway) is controlled by the motor cortex and the sensory cortex in the brain, and it extends through the medulla which sends the motor impulse downward through the spinal column. If this pathway gets obstructed, it may cause spinal muscles to tighten. This may cause the sympathetic nerves to become blocked, in turn, causing impulse problems.

For example, with liver cancer, we can find that the right-hand-side of T9 has a blockage or is tight. This can be a result of the motor cortex or sensory cortex in the left side of the brain getting blocked. So when we check the blockage, we should pay attention to the brain's motor cortex and sensory cortex on the *opposite* side.

Can the Vascular System Cause Cancer?

Another factor that may cause cancer is the vascular system. We know the blood carries oxygen and nutrition to all parts of the body to supply the cells and organs. If the vessels have a function problem, it may cause an oxygen and blood circulation problem which could lead to a variety of organ cancers.

Most vessel problems are found in the arteries, which may get blocked due to high cholesterol, so we try to lower cholesterol in the diet in order to prevent heart disease and blood pressure problems.

To prevent arterial blockages, doctors concentrate on protein and cholesterol in their patients' diets, but calcium needs attention as well—it can initiate a blockage which could cause prostate cancer. According to medical studies, high levels of calcium may block the kidneys and smaller arteries, causing the local area to experience poor blood supply and low oxygen—these relate to cell mutation and can cause cancer.

Other major vessels are located on the spinal cord, and little attention is paid to them. The Spinal Artery has two branches—the anterior spinal artery and the posterior spinal artery. The anterior spinal artery supplies the anterior portion of the spinal cord. The posterior spinal artery arises from the vertebral artery, adjacent to the medulla oblongata

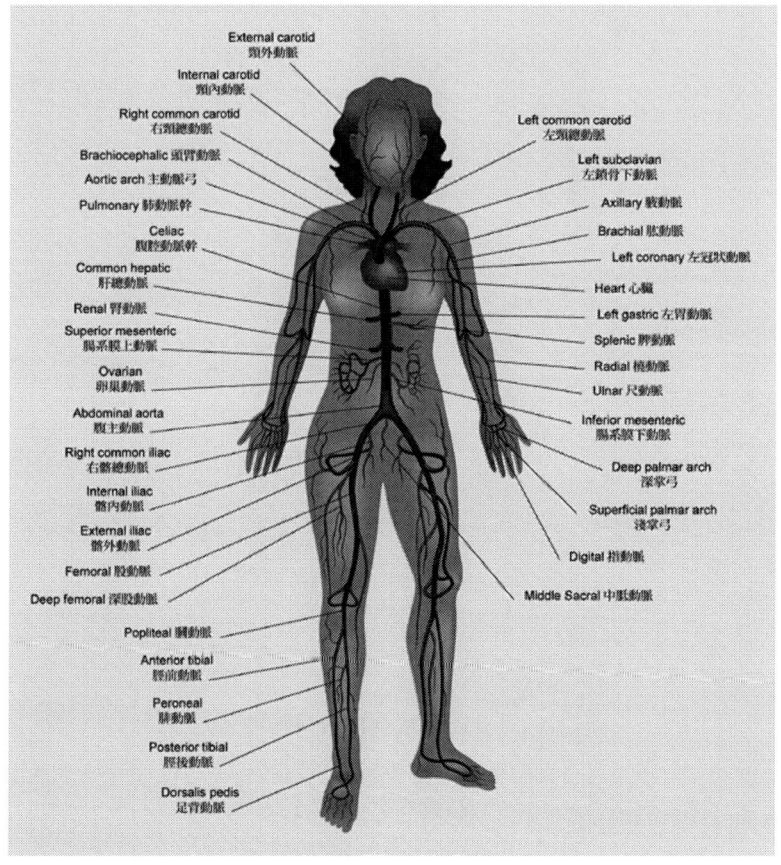

Anterior spinal arterial stroke can be caused by an interruption of the blood supply in the anterior spinal artery, affecting sensation, motor control, and bowel control. The severity of the disorder depends on the exact location of the defect and how long it persists. Symptoms may improve to varying degrees once the blood supply returns to normal.

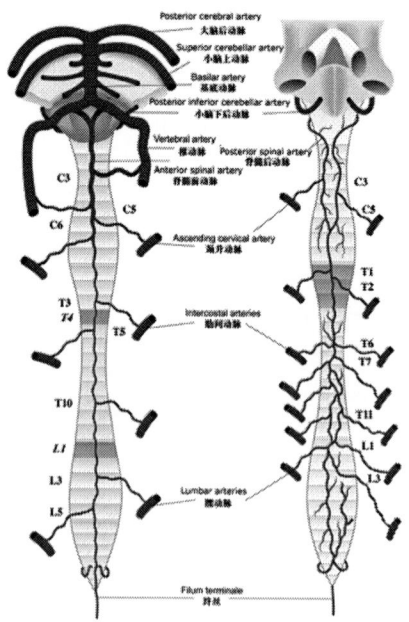

Spinal Artery

Even though the spinal cord plays a major role in the functioning of every organ in the body, little, if any, attention is paid to these arteries which control the oxygen level reaching the spinal cord. Because the spinal arteries originate from the neck area, tension in that area may constrict blood flow to the spinal artery. This indicates that exercising the neck area is important to treating cancer. Much of Chi Gong exercise focuses the movement on the neck area, such as the movement called Opening the Sky Door.

What about Mineral Supplements?

In an effort to prevent bone loss, many people in America take huge amounts of calcium supplements, believing that the kidneys will flush any excess from their bodies. This is true, but only in the short term. Taking a daily overdose of calcium (or any mineral) over a long period of time will cause the kidneys to overload and may result in kidney problems. In recent medical studies, it was discovered that taking too much calcium can cause prostate cancer.

Why is the overuse of calcium a cause for concern? In the Tom Tam Healing System, it is easy to see the connection between calcium levels and prostate cancer, because the kidney and prostate are connected, and the blockages in the lumbar are adjacent to one another—the kidney's energy point is located at L2 and the prostate's is on L3.

When L2 is blocked, L3 may be blocked as well. Another difficulty, that is often overlooked, is the possible link between calcium supplementation and ovarian and uterine cancers (though, to date, I have found no scientific studies to confirm this).

Arteries of Systemic Circulation

Multivitamin supplementation may also be linked to some cancers. Research from the National Cancer Institute reported that men who take too many multivitamins may be increasing their risk of dying from prostate cancer. Taking a multivitamin more than seven times a week was associated with a 30% increased risk of advanced prostate cancer and a doubling of the risk of death from the disease in the study.

Many cancer patients enjoy taking vitamin C for healing, yet vitamin C supplementation may interfere with chemotherapy. A 2008 study from Memorial Sloan-Kettering Cancer Center found that vitamin C was absorbed by cancer cells and protected those cells from chemotherapy drugs.

Remember, don't believe the hypothesis that the more supplements you take, the more likely you will prevent or heal cancer. You should ask your doctor or do your own research before taking any supplements. I am not against taking supplements, but a deficiency needs to be confirmed through a simple medical checkup before taking them.

There are countless factors which can cause cancer, but the most important is oxygen. In any healing system, the first step in correcting the problem may have to do with oxygen supply to the affected cells—we must discover where the blockage is so we can benefit more people.

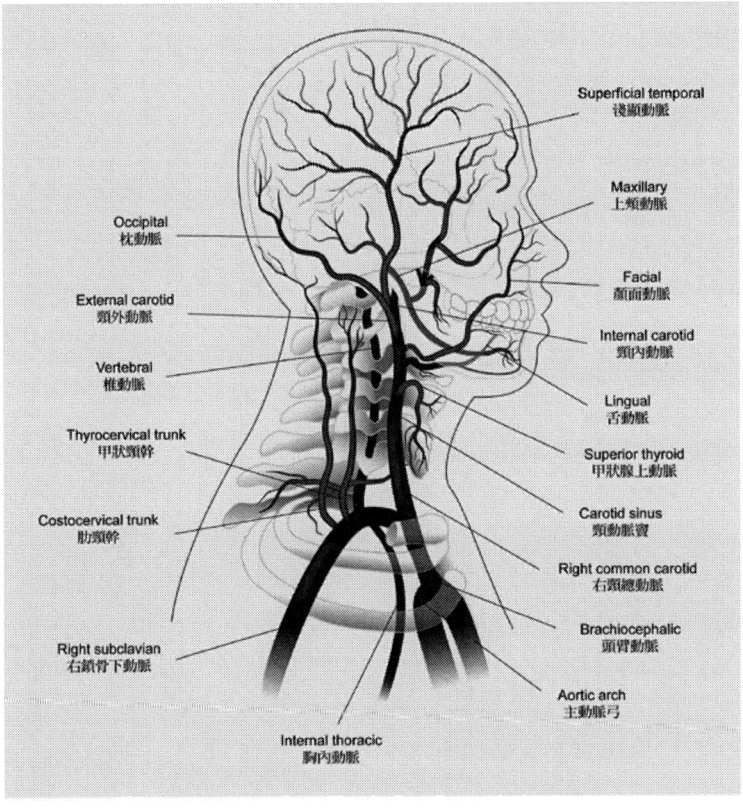

Arteries of Right Side Head and Neck

How Does Diet Fit In?

When they receive the initial cancer diagnosis, some patients will blame their diet or possibly a vitamin or mineral deficiency, and often will want to change their diet as an approach to healing their cancer. There are many theories about this approach and most of the dietary changes focus on eliminating the intake of chemicals and meat.

Depending on where you look or whom you talk to, just about anything around us has been blamed for causing cancer: pollution in our food and air, water with added chemicals, environmental pollutants, and much more. All of these complaints are related to chemicals.

Many experts try to uncover the 'secrets' of the chemical causes of cancer, which is sad. They waste so much time and money in support of studies that cannot explain or prove which food might be responsible. Many vegetarians have cancer; newborn babies who are only fed mother's milk get cancer; nutritionists and diet experts get cancer while following specific diets aimed at preventing it.

Other experts follow the Warburg effect theory about pH balance because alkaline and acid levels are easy to evaluate through laboratory testing, and the theory is gaining in popularity. In this theory, testing can detect a pH level which can be compared with a 'normal' range. The body has the ability to balance its acidity and maintain its pH within a normal and healthy range from 7.35 to 7.45, but if the patient's pH is outside this range, many experts advise their patients to change their diet to bring their pH back in line. Any product containing chemicals, in addition to food, can affect the pH level in the body.

Exercise and increased respiration can change the pH without any food intake. When we are doing any aerobic exercise, our breathing and exhalation cause an exchange of carbon dioxide. Rapid breathing causes a release of more carbon dioxide and this can raise the pH to become more alkaline and less acidic.

The Future of Cancer Research

Researchers are always in search of new ideas. Scientists, especially, should never be afraid to try anything, even what might appear to be a 'stupid' idea. If this stupid idea can end up saving a million lives suffering from cancer, should it be tried? Why not? Maybe someday a medical researcher or medical doctor will put a laser beam on an acupuncture model for ten minutes accidentally, instead of using radiation directly on their patient and discover the beneficial results firsthand.

Clinical trials evaluate new ways to treat cancer, and are an option for many lung cancer patients. In some case studies, all patients receive the new treatment or newly developed drug. In another method, doctors compare therapies by giving the new treatment to one group of patients and the standard therapy to a different group. However, the studies are defined and limited by Western medical methods and theory exclusively.

Unfortunately, 50 years of study still seem to net the same results. How many patients die from their cancer during or after these clinical trials? We cannot say that the trials themselves cause death, but we *should* question whether the trials are safe. I hope and advise all of my patients to ask this question of their doctors before they consent to participate in trials: "Is it safe for me to be a guinea pig?"

Preventing Cancer

Do Supplements Have a Place in Cancer Prevention?

People often favor vitamin C supplements or orange juice over eating an actual orange. In fact, after a diagnosis of colon cancer, a high percentage of patients double or even triple, their mineral and juice intake. Advertisements of mineral products state that food from the grocery is missing something important that causes mineral deficiency and will, in turn, lead to illness. They repeat this message again and again until it is deeply imbedded in our subconscious. This creates fear and then, when an illness arises, the subconscious sends out that stored signal stating "we need some kind of mineral." The fear hidden in the memory can cause a psychological dependency and addiction even if we already have sufficient minerals and vitamins in our bodies.

In my practice, I have a treatment to help addicted patients stop using vitamins, minerals, and juice. If we can get rid of the vitamin pills and juice, and eat the actual fruit instead, it will guarantee a decrease in digestion problems. But how many people will make this simple, but important, change?

A Cancer-Preventing Diet

Most experts believe that a good diet may prevent colorectal cancer. Here is what experts at the National Cancer Institute recommend:

"20 to 30 grams of fiber a day. Good sources: Whole-grain breads, cereals and pastas, beans, brown rice, and plenty of fruits and vegetables—at least five servings a day. Limit fat to 30 percent of daily caloric intake, with no more than 10 percent coming from saturated fats like butter and coconut and palm oils.

"New research suggests that calcium and folic acid may contribute to the prevention of colorectal cancer as well. Good sources of calcium include skim or low-fat milk and dairy products, broccoli, kale, salmon, and sardines with bones. Folic acid can be found in fortified cereals, dark green leafy vegetables, some nuts and seeds, and dried beans."

After we read this recommendation, these new questions arise: can this diet prevent colitis and constipation, and can it stop the growth of polyps? If it cannot help with colitis and constipation, how can it prevent or heal colorectal cancer? In our experience, we know that if patients have colitis, they should not have dairy products, which includes any type of milk. Even mother's milk, though good for a baby, is not good for a grown man.

In my commonsense diet developed from my practice, I advise patients to eat everything, but in moderation. Especially when the patient receives surgery, chemo, and radiation, they need more red meat to replace blood cells. The best is beef stew or chicken soup; they are easy to eat and easily digested.

In my diet system, liquids are the worst things, and their consumption should be monitored. Soups, however, usually contain an ingredient that requires chewing—this stimulates digestion—so soups and stews are *not* considered liquids. The greater the liquid intake, the harder the large intestine will have to work. Another reason to limit liquids is because there are too many chemicals added to them. Soda, especially diet varieties, juice, too much coffee, and too much beer are bad, also.

A good diet is simple: eat more meat and vegetables. This is called "yin and yang balance."

Exercise as a Cancer Preventative

Exercise is another doctor's suggestion for the prevention of colorectal cancer. Studies suggest that "regular physical activity cuts colon cancer risk practically in half, but there is no evidence of a similar protection against rectal cancer." Colorectal cancer occurs mainly in people over 50. During middle age, back problems are the most frequent complaints, not cancer. When people are over 50, they should do easy exercise and avoid weightlifting because weightlifting can compress the spinal column, which, in turn, may develop a blockage.

When exercising, we should direct attention to the neck area where the vagus nerve and phrenic nerve are found. The neck exercise is easy, simply stretch or turn the head to the left and then to the right. Tension in the neck area is especially common in people who work with computers, so this exercise is especially important for them.

Preventing Colorectal Cancer

If we want to prevent colorectal cancer effectively, the first thing we need to do is keep the intestines functioning normally. Proper diet, whether influenced by the West or East, is one way to keep the intestines working easily and healthily. Medicines and minerals can heal the problem temporarily, but cannot treat the root of the problem.

In the Tom Tam Healing System, any problem with the function of the large or small intestine means there is a blockage around the T11 area. So far, diet, medication, and exercise aren't enough to help digestive problems such as colitis and Crohn's disease or constipation (both of which are conditions which cause inflammation of the lining and wall of the bowel). But, in my healing system, using any technique to open the blockage will make the digestion problem disappear.

So my belief system for colorectal cancer prevention or healing is to open blockages rather than focus on diet and exercise. Of course, diet and exercise are important but, in the digestion system, I believe that the opening of blockages is *more* important.

Scientists believe that colorectal cancer may result from cell overgrowth when new cells are generated to replace the diseased tissue. But why does this happen? No one has the answer. But I find one thing in common with all bowel problems: they have the same blockage from T10 to T12 in the thoracic part of the spine. Most colon cancer patients have a blockage in T11 or T12 on the left side, and those with rectal cancer have one around the sacrum area. For some, it can be around the lumbar area.

The intestine is long, so the blockage location depends on which part of the intestine is experiencing a problem. Therefore, the blockage is not at a single, fixed point; it varies on the lower spinal column. Don't let this confuse you. When we look for the blockage in the spinal column, visually we will see the blockage as a puffing or swelling, as a different skin color or tone, or as a mole around that area. Sometimes we will see a curvature of the spinal column as scoliosis.

We can open this blockage with many techniques, such as Tui Na, acupuncture, or using massage tools—any stimulation can decrease the blockage. During treatment to the blockage area, a patient may feel the intestines move. This means the intestines are functioning and, when they function, bioelectricity can get through better because nerve resistance has decreased.

In my Tong Ren healing class, many participants have colorectal cancer and most are classified as stage IV. I'm proud to say that our healing rate is high in these cases. Some colorectal cancer patients use chemo, radiation and surgery, but some receive no treatment from their doctors.

When we treat colorectal cancer, it is necessary to pay close attention to the vagus nerve where the acupuncture point LI18 is located. Also stimulate and open the blockage in the pathway of the phrenic nerve where point LI17 is located. Furthermore, in cases where the cancer has spread to the liver, we should treat the T9 and ST21 points, also. In addition, if the cancer has spread to the lung, we should treat that as a secondary cancer and use T3 and CV17.

Since many experts believe, without doubt, that bowel problems are connected to the consumption of a diet high in fat and low in fiber, research naturally focuses on diet for colon and rectal cancers.

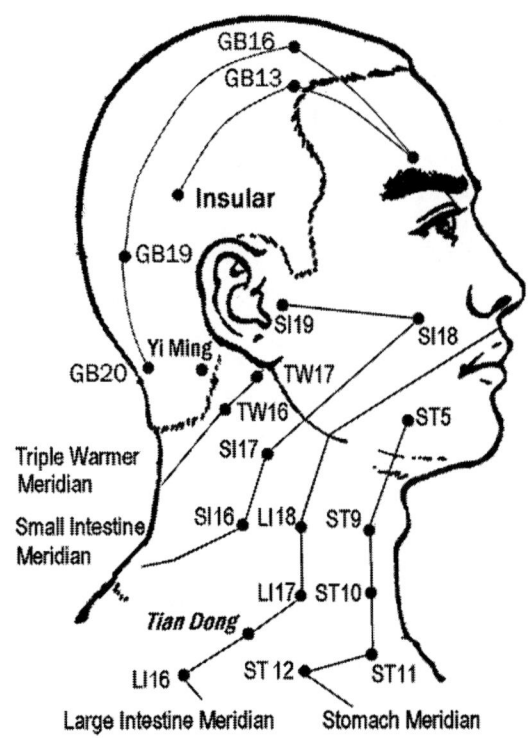

LI17 and LI18

In fact, the topic of diet in America is a highly charged subject of discussion—more so than anywhere else in the world. There are many diet books, diet systems, and cultural eating diversities in this country, yet diet cannot stop colon cancer, weight problems, or digestive problems such as stomach ulcers, constipation, inflammatory bowel diseases, chronic ulcerative colitis, or Crohn's disease.

Despite the high number of nutritionists in this country, weight problems and other diet-related problems still exist and are increasing. Why? Because confusion results due to the vast number of different diet theories as well as to advertising by companies hoping to profit from Americans' obsession with diet.

Healing Cancer

Misguided Treatments for Healing Cancer

Many doctors, when treating cancer, advise their patients to get more fresh air or practice deep breathing in order to increase their oxygen levels. They also often advise their patients to use aerobic exercise to increase their heart's capacity to pump blood, which in turn increases lung capacity. But many cancer patients are too weak to exercise because of their disease or because of side effects from chemo, radiation, or surgery. Relaxation is more important for these patients than aerobic exercise. For them, deep breathing exercises can help heal their cancer, but breathing exercises alone rarely heal cancer.

Some doctors believe that overeating causes oxygen deficiency, so they advise their patients to eat smaller, nutrient-dense meals and stop eating junk food. Other experts advise patients to take vitamins or supplements to heal or prevent cancer. We often see cancer patients taking dozens of vitamin or mineral supplements, though studies show that an overdose of certain minerals and vitamins can cause side effects. Some believe that vitamin F can increase the oxygen-carrying capacity of hemoglobin in red blood cells...yet how many of these patients are healed or survive?

An intestinal cleansing method is used by many patients in an attempt to heal their cancer. Cleaning poison from affected organs is beneficial to general health, but cancer is a condition of oxygen deficiency. How can cleansing of the intestines, or any other organ, change the level of oxygen within the body? This is a misguided approach to healing cancer.

Using supplementary oxygen from sources such as oxygenated drinking water, fresh foods and juices, magnesium peroxide, and magnesium dioxide also have been suggested by some doctors. Some systems even believe that bathing in oxygenated water can heal cancer.

In China, the breathing practices of Chi Gong and Tai Chi—as well as those of the Indian system called Yoga—are intended to increase oxygen within the body. These are called internal exercises, and no doubt can help in healing cancer, but the healing rate percentage is low. Does the internal exercise increase the intake of oxygen or just correct the organ's function and ability to process the oxygen? There is a need for scientific study to answer these questions.

When a doctor suggests that any particular therapy is effective for healing cancer, a patient may try it without question. For this reason, no matter what method is being contemplated, its healing rate must be considered before making recommendations.

Drug Companies and Doctors Focus on the Wrong Areas

Throughout the world, much attention and investment is focused on the *chemical* treatment of cancer. Over the last 50 years, however, the healing rate of cancer has remained the same; many people still die from cancer or chemotherapy's side effects. So it appears as though cancer experts are not learning from their experiences—they continue to develop new drugs in collaboration with pharmaceutical companies. Huge amounts of money are being invested in developing chemicals for use in the Warburg Effect study.

Sadly, this demonstrates that pharmaceutical companies are interested only in *drug research*, not in the *healing benefits* of the oxygen which is freely available all around us. A high percentage of cancer patients participate in their clinical trials, making them human guinea pigs for the drug makers...but at what cost and for what benefit?

As scientists throughout the world pay more attention to Warburg's research about cancer cells fermenting sugar, drug companies attempt to profit from the idea. On December 21, 2009, the *Boston Globe* reported that, *"In the 1920s, the German scientist Otto Warburg first observed that cancer cells burn sugar differently than normal cells do...Finding ways to disrupt metabolism is the idea behind Agios Pharmaceuticals, a Cambridge company co founded by Cantley that last year raised $33 million. And in September, the American Association for Cancer Research hosted a four-day meeting focusing on cancer and metabolism. Last week, the journal* Science *named cancer metabolism an area to watch in 2010."*

Some studies show that the cancer cell's glycolysis is a result of a metabolism problem. Researchers, however, are focusing on using the immune system to kill cancerous cells, not on the metabolic system, which is used to mutate the cell back to a normal condition. Why are they doing this?

Other studies concentrate on the use of external oxygen sources to balance the body's internal oxygen—but a low-oxygen problem originates from *within* our organs, not from *external* factors. If an internal organ dysfunctions while taking in oxygen, it doesn't matter how much oxygen we add, the organ still has functional problems. Doctors attempt to use a variety of methods to increase oxygen to different parts of the body, but few seem interested in correcting the body's *use* of oxygen.

'Healing' products are continually being developed for profit, rather than for healing—and, sadly, many patients believe the advertising claims.

The Diaphragm is Unique

Have you ever heard of diaphragm cancer? It is a very interesting medical phenomenon, though I have never heard anyone ask this question. The diaphragm cannot get primary cancer, yet it *can* get secondary cancer from other organs. The secondary cancer cannot be called 'diaphragm cancer', so do not be confused.

So why do humans never have diaphragm cancer? When we search the Internet, we find that no one can provide an answer, and there is no interesting research about diaphragm cancer.

In my understanding, cancer is caused by a blockage in the spinal column where the sympathetic nerve is located. [Remember that the sympathetic nervous system is part of the autonomic nervous system.] The diaphragm doesn't have an autonomic nerve, but rather, it has its own independent nerve system including the phrenic nerve and accessory phrenic nerve.

Another interesting phenomenon: only humans and mammals have diaphragms (and the phrenic nerve to control it), and only humans and mammals get cancer. Non-mammal beings—such as fish, birds and insects—do not get cancer (though there is some debate as to whether it actually does exist other than as a rarity). So some might wonder if a mammal's milk causes cancer, but the jury is still out on that issue.

Focus on the Diaphragm for Healing

Many experts focus all their attention on diet to prevent or heal cancer. They watch the acid and alkaline, pH and enzymes, vitamins and minerals. We know that when oxygen levels change, all biochemistries are going to change (this even happens with metal, as it can be oxidized also). We pay too much attention to diet and chemical balance—now is the time to change this and turn our attention to the diaphragm as a way to heal cancer.

The phrenic nerve is long: from C3, C4, and C5 to the diaphragm in the abdomen. Opening the blockage for the phrenic nerve plays an important part in healing cancer. We must identify the blockage that is causing the phrenic nerve's function problem—it is mainly on the LI17 area and then ST 11 where it is located under LI17.

Every human being has a phrenic nerve, but not all have the accessory phrenic nerve. Statistics show that 48 percent of Chinese have the accessory phrenic nerve and 52 percent of Americans have it.

Why do some people have this nerve while others don't? We can determine what percentage of cancer patients have the accessory phrenic nerve, and consider whether this relates to the incidence of cancer.

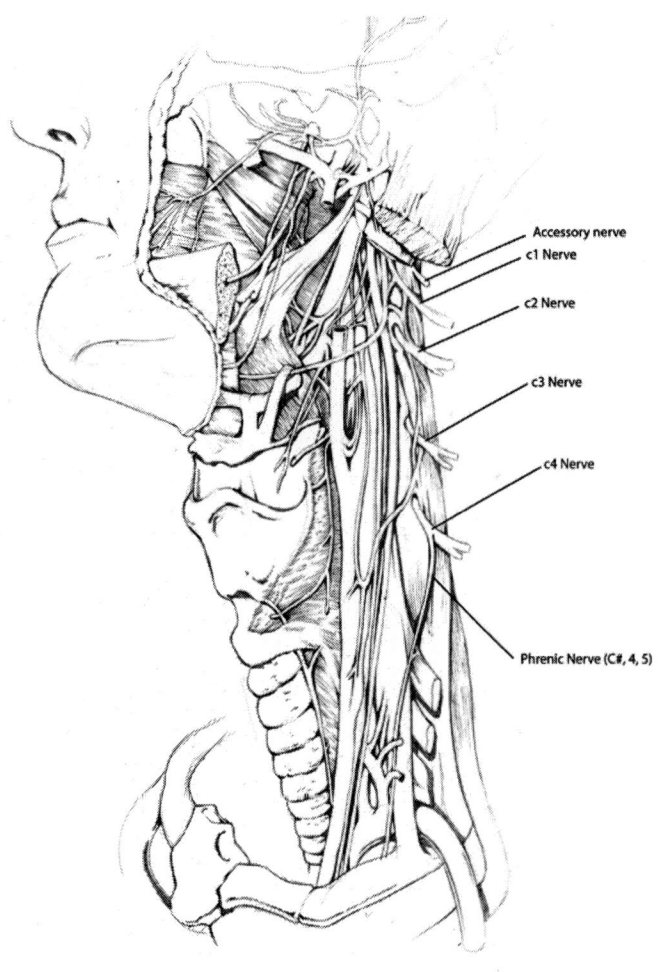

Bioelectricity's Role in Healing Cancer

We know that a healthy body depends upon healthy cells. Healthy cells function like efficient power plants based on two types of energy sources: biochemical and bioelectric.

We know that the maturation of cancer cells is connected with the biochemical function. Chemical healing methods are used throughout the world in different forms. Chemotherapy, which is very common in the US, is not widely used in China, so when people there are diagnosed with cancer, many look to using herbs for healing. But, in fact, herbs and diet are considered chemical forms of healing, because any material (including air and water) that goes into the body is 'chemical.'

Because cancer can be caused when the impulse from the brain (which needs to pass to the medulla and then to the organ through the nerves) is blocked, bioelectricity provides an additional approach to healing. This new concept in healing, which is gaining attention in China, is based on the stimulation of meridian and acupuncture points, yet its healing effects have been limited.

In China, the bioelectricity theory is mainly used to support the practice and philosophy of Chi Gong, and it is not separated from the meridian philosophy. In Traditional Chinese Medicine, meridians are simply a path for Chi, or energy. The meridian system does not equate to the nervous system—the nervous system can be seen, but the meridian system is an abstract concept that cannot be seen by any modern high-tech equipment.

Bioelectricity was not discovered through Chinese medicine—an Italian medical doctor, Luigi Galvani (September 9, 1737 – December 4, 1798) made the discovery. In 1771, Galvani discovered that the muscles of dead frogs twitched when struck by a spark. This was one of the first forays into the study of bioelectricity, a field that studies the electrical patterns and signals of the nervous system.

In Western medical practice, only the impulse and chemical synapse of the nerve appear to be of interest. There is little interest in bioelectricity and most medical experts are not knowledgeable about it.

Scientists have proven that bioelectricity exists in the body. Each cell in the body, in any tissue or organism, has bioelectricity, or electromagnetic fields. These include the cell membrane potential and the electric currents that flow through nerves and muscles as a result of action potentials. Biological cells use bioelectricity to store metabolic energy, to do work or trigger internal changes, and to signal one another.

Bioelectromagnetism is an aspect of all living things, including all plants and animals. Some animals have acute bioelectromagnetic sensors. For example, migratory birds are believed to navigate in part by sensing the Earth's magnetic field. Where there is bio-current, there must be voltage (V) and resistance (R). This concept is from Ohm's law, which is: **I = V/R**, where **I** is the current through the resistance in units of amperes, **V** is the potential difference measured across the resistance in units of volts, and **R** is the resistance of the conductor in units of ohms. More specifically, Ohm's law states that the *R* in this relation is constant, independent of the current .

In Ohm's law, we understand that if there is a current and voltage, there must be a conductor. Identified only as Chi pathways, the meridians of TCM cannot be conductors. However, it is easy to check the nervous system for bioelectrical current and voltage because nerves—which are the pathways for impulses *from* the brain or feedback *to* the brain—are the conductors. So, if nerves are conductors, then when a nerve is in low resistance, bioelectricity passes easily. If the resistance is zero, called the super conductor, then we can be 'superman.'

The TCM system cannot use Ohm's law, because the voltage or resistor cannot be found in the meridian.

If a nerve has high resistance, then the bio-current will be low even if the voltage remains at the same level and the cells, tissues, or organisms will function poorly. Through medical studies, scientists have ascertained that cancer cells carry a low voltage of bioelectricity. Western medicine rarely, if ever, considers resistance in the nervous system, because it does not have a technique to find it.

When people become sick, bioelectricity is rarely accessed for healing. If a patient has a biochemical problem, it is treated with herbs, drugs, or diet. If they have a problem with a *bioelectrical* function, *biochemical* agents are still prescribed—but why? Pharmaceutical companies and medical doctors show no interest in the use of bioelectricity for healing—it is not taught in Western medical schools and it is rare to find any information about it.

The Spinal Column's Role in Healing Cancer

Many healing systems have developed their own way of understanding how the spinal column connects to an internal organ. The Tom Tam Healing System has its own understanding that is distinct from the others.

To heal any type of cancer or tumor, we must open the blockage on the spinal column. The Tom Tam Healing System, based on 20 years of experience in my practice, involves detecting the Ouch point related to a blockage. These Ouch points (also called energy blockage points) are detectable by anyone, and detection is repeatable. Around the Ouch point on the spinal area, the skin or spinal column is abnormal, such as the skin's color, a mole, rash, spinal curvature, swelling, or muscular tension.

The first step toward healing is to confirm a doctor's diagnosis regarding which organ is cancerous. Next, follow that diagnosis to find the location of the blockage on the spinal column which is related to the cancer. The diagnosis is a medical doctor's job; our job is to find the blockage to prove that the cancer does, indeed, exist. The next step is to heal the cancer.

Remember: a blockage on the spinal column does not indicate cancer, but when there is a medically confirmed cancer diagnosis, we can *always* find a related blockage. The blockage itself is never used as a diagnosis for cancer, because that may mislead and unnecessarily traumatize the patient.

If the body is in a low-oxygen condition but does not have any blockage on the spinal cord, cancer cannot form—the condition will manifest itself in a different way, such as low energy level or shortness of breath.

The blockage on the spinal area may be the primary cause of the cancer, but we also need to consider other factors, like the function of the phrenic nerve, the accessory phrenic nerve, growth hormone, medulla and blood circulation.

In Tong Ren healing, we can use GB12, TW16, TW17, and Tian Dong to release tension on the neck and free the blockage of the spinal artery. Benefits from doing this are not limited to healing cancer—keeping the artery in good condition and free from blockage is important for healing any disease. For instance, in the case of brain cancer, we need to pay close attention to blood circulation in the brain.

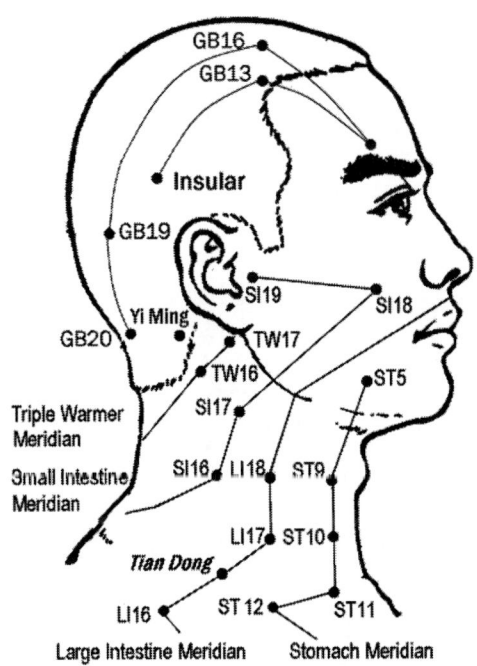

Central Nervous System and Bladder Meridian

The Role of Chi in Healing Cancer

Many experts, Western medical professionals, and especially the so-called Skeptics, deny or even laugh at the concept of using Chi for healing the body. It is interesting how people have no problem believing in Einstein's theories on energy, $E=mc^2$, but are reluctant to accept the notion of Chi. Different cultures have different names for Chi, but it does not matter what you call it—Chi exists and it usually circulates throughout the body along various meridians.

In my healing theory, I often use the word *bioelectricity* because this energy force can be tested and measured in the body. Bioelectricity is measured by the impulse that passes through the nervous system. Yet if we limit the practice of healing to only the Chi, we often cannot explain or understand the movement of healing throughout the body. The experience of Chi passing along the meridian cannot be denied, however, if we use only the nervous system to explain the movement of Chi, we will get confused.

Locating Blockage Points for Use in Healing

In cancer treatment, we can easily find the blockage on the patient's spinal column where the sympathetic nerve is located. When we press the blockage area, the patient may feel pain and muscular tension. We must open this blockage to allow bioelectricity to flow more freely. If we use the bladder meridian points on the skull, it may make the spinal blockage easier to open.

The bladder meridian has four major meridian points on the skull: BL6, BL7, BL8, and BL9. When these points are stimulated, an impulse may be created which travels to the opposite side of the body. In the clinical practice for healing, I often use these four bladder meridian points to help open the blockage.

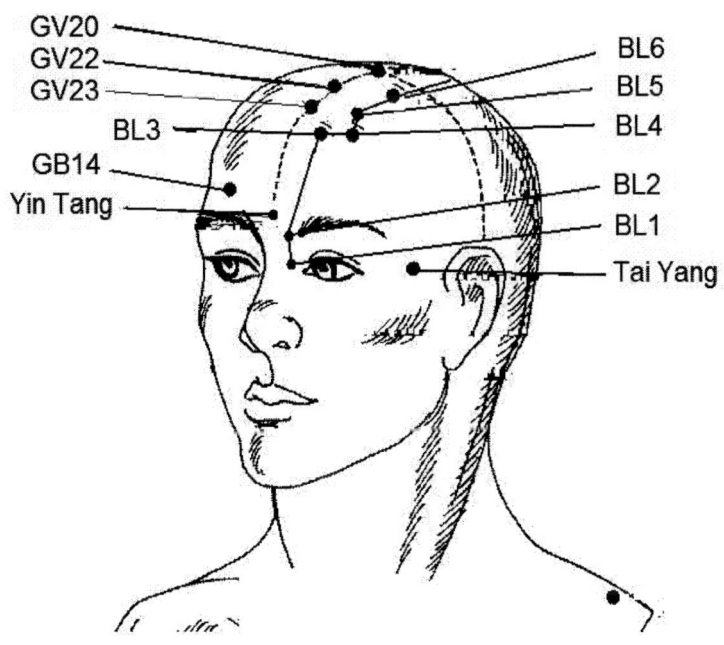

BL6 is called Cheng Guang in Chinese, which means "Receive Light." In TCM, BL6 is for healing headaches, nasal obstruction, and blurry vision. It is located on the head, 2.5 cun posterior to the anterior hairline, 1.3 cun lateral to the midline, which is the governing vessel meridian.

In the Tom Tam Healing System, we believe that BL6 and GV22 are the major hormone reflex points. When children are diagnosed with any genetic problem, we can see a big improvement in healing by using GV22 and BL6. Because BL6 is related to hormone function, stimulating it can balance the hormones.

BL7 is called Tong Tian, which means "Connecting to the Sky." It is located 4 cun posterior to anterior hairline, and 1.5 cun lateral to the midline of the head. In TCM, BL7 is used to treat headache, dizziness, hemiplegia, mouth deviation, respiratory disorders, nasal congestion, and nosebleed. BL7 is located around the motor cortex area, meaning when we stimulate this point, it can affect the body's motor nervous system.

For example, when a patient is diagnosed with Sarcoma in the arm or leg, we can find the "Ouch point" on BL7 on the opposite side on the skull. In my practice, this point is a major point for healing problems with arm and leg movement, such as MS, stroke, and arthritis.

BL8 is around the sensory cortex and association cortex in the brain, which is called Luo Que. It is 1.5 cun posterior to BL7. In TCM, this point helps calm the mind and clear the sense organs. Sensory nerves gather information from the environment, send that information to the spinal cord, and speed the message to the brain.

The brain makes sense of that message and fires off a response, and then motor neurons deliver the instruction impulse to the rest of the body. The spinal cord simply acts like a bundle of cables, enabling the signals to travel along the spine, to and from the brain, at all times.

BL8 is a point rarely used in TCM—instead, in the Tom Tam Healing System, it is preferably used for treating sensory cortex or motor cortex problems, rather than using GV20. The brain's cerebrum has right and left hemispheres, which are separated by the longitudinal fissure.

When the cerebrum has a problem, it normally occurs in the hemispheres (and less often in the longitudinal fissure where the GV meridian passes through). If the patient had a stroke, it is in one hemisphere, on the rear of the longitudinal fissure.

The corpus callosum is one of the two main connections between the two hemispheres of the brain. The job of the corpus callosum is to route communication between the two hemispheres. Yet when people have a corpus callosum-related problem, it is usually more involved in one side or the other than in the middle.

A sensory cortex problem is not easy to treat. For example, Complex Regional Pain Syndrome (CRPS), also known as Reflex Sympathetic Dystrophy (RSD), is a chronic neurological syndrome. Western medicine struggles to treat RSD because it does not understand how to use the sensory cortex for healing. When we stimulate the BL8 and GV19, it results in good healing.

BL9 (Yu Zhen), also called Jade Pillow in TCM, is located near the medulla oblongata, vision cortex and cerebellum area. BL9 is in the occipital region, in a depression 1.5 cun lateral to the superior aspect of the external occipital protuberance.

In TCM, this point is often forgotten, though it can be used to heal eye pain, visual disturbances (but not problems with the eyeballs or eye nerve), myopia tension, heaviness of the head or neck, headache, and vertigo. In my practice, this is a common point to balance the heart, lung, and vessel problems. It is a reflex point for the medulla.

The medulla is sometimes called the Life Center. We very seldom hear of a patient having a problem with the medulla itself, because Western medical practice focuses on the tumor that can grow in the medulla oblongata area, not on the organ's function or blockage.

BL10 (Tian Zhu), called Sky Pillar in TCM, is located between GV15 and GB20, at the level between cervical vertebrae C1 and C2. BL10 is another seldom-used point in acupuncture, but in the Tom Tam Healing System, it is a beginning point for the spinal cord and the connection point for the opposite of BL9.

In TCM theory, BL10 connects to the same side of BL9 for the Chi's pass channel. In my theory, the Chi runs from the right side of BL10 to the left side of BL9, on the opposite side of the spinal cord. In practice, we need to pay attention to this point, because it is located near the C1 and C2 area, where it can easily become blocked from emotional or physical tension.

Western medicine has much knowledge about the central nervous system, but that does not mean they know how to use this knowledge to treat problems caused by it. TCM does not have knowledge about the central nervous system, but has much experience in treating related problems.

If we could combine Western knowledge of medical anatomy with Eastern knowledge of Chi, methods of medical stimulation, and healing experience, then we could cure many difficult and otherwise 'incurable' diseases.

BL1 is called Jīng Míng (Bright Eyes) and is located on the face, in the depression superior to the inner canthus. This meridian point automatically heals eye problems.

Also on the face, **BL2** is called Cuan Zhu (Bamboo Gathering), and is located above BL1 on the medial end of the eyebrow. It is no doubt that this point can help heal eye problems.

BL1 and BL2 are close to the acupuncture point, Yin Tang, which is the 'third eye.' It is located on the forehead, midway between the medial ends of the two eyebrows. In my healing practice, I often use Yin Tang for relaxation. In the Chakra system, this area of the body is the 6th Chakra, Brow, or "mind center" and in TCM it is referred to as "Calms the Spirit."

The forebrain is separated into two sides, right and left—BL1 and BL2 only affect the left side. Using BL1 and BL2 is more direct and effective for healing the forebrain than the Yin Tang, which is in the middle. Besides healing eye problems and calming the mind, BL1 and BL2 can help with attention dysfunction such as ADD and ADHD and blurry mind.

The bladder meridian has points **BL3**, **BL4**, and **BL5** on the forehead. These points can be used for healing the mind, emotions, addiction, memory, trauma or any psychological problem, which is important in treating cancer patients. Some patients may experience fear, anger, or even suicidal thoughts, which are in the hypothalamus—we can stimulate BL6 and GV22 to help.

In the Tom Tam Healing System, bone marrow has its blockage point in **T1**. With any disease related to anemia or a blood disorder, we can find the blockage in the T1 area.

Melanoma and sarcoma are difficult to treat using Western medicine, because these cancers are secondary, not primary. Though Western medicine does not know where the primary cancer originates, in Tong Ren healing we can find the common point and blockage in the **T4** area. Skin cancer also has its blockage in T4, because it is the sweat gland function, which releases toxins through the skin.

A point used on the doll is **K27**, then we follow the kidney meridian down to the chest, stomach, leg, and bottom of the foot at the location of K1. When we use the hammer to stimulate the kidney meridian, a patient may feel warmth or heat from the face moving down to the chest, then the stomach and finally down toward the leg as oxygen or Chi is moving along that path. Using this method to open the kidney meridian, the patient can feel much release from both physical and psychological symptoms.

Using These Points to Heal Cancer

For healing cancer, we must first calm the patient and release their psychological problems using **BL1** to **BL5**.

We adjust the growth hormone that can affect growth of new cells by using **BL6**.

BL7 and **BL8** can lower resistance along the meridians by eliminating tension in the back.

With **BL9**, we can build up more energy from circulation in the lungs, heart, and vessels.

BL10 can be used to give the skull more support and increase circulation.

Below **BL11**, I use the Huatuojiaji points for more effective healing. These points are closer to the spinal column than the back Shu points along the bladder meridian.

The West and East's medical arguments are focused on the meridians and Chi, and on acupuncture points. In the Tom Tam Healing System, I realize the value of each and use both as I concentrate on healing results rather than theory.

Diet and Cancer Healing

During the practice of Chinese Chi Gong or Tai Chi Chuan exercises, the mind and body relax while breathing slows down. This type of internal exercise can release less carbon dioxide and lower pH. After external exercise, many people become short on oxygen and experience shallow breathing. However, after internal exercises, people will feel the Dantian has been filled with a lot of Chi and oxygen and their pH is more balanced, without any food intake.

Tests to determine pH are taken from saliva, urine, and blood, but the pH level of saliva and urine are in constant flux—diet, internal and external exercises, even emotions can cause a change to pH. The body works hard to keep its pH balanced, but it is nearly impossible to achieve, and maintain, a high-alkaline pH for a prolonged period.

Many special-diet healing strategies believe that poor diet can cause cancer, but this is counter to the understanding expressed in the Warburg effect. According to Warburg's study, cancer cannot exist in an alkaline environment. The factors that cause alkaline levels to go up or down are something pH experts do not appear to consider in relation to cancer.

In the West, the diet logically divides into two types: alkaline and acid, or 'good' and 'bad.' The Chinese diet also has two types—Yin food and Yang food—but does not label them good or bad. TCM theory has five elements, each balanced and related to the others.

In the West, after being diagnosed with cancer, many people will stop eating red meat and sugar, believing that they cause cancer. In China, when a cancer patient loses weight, they eat *more* red meat and sugar to replace the calories and protein lost during treatment. In the West, there are vast amounts of advice from experts about using diet to heal cancer. Each one has its own idea and philosophy, yet how many cancer patients do we see healed from these special diets?

In TCM, most patients learn from a young age the importance of diet in healing the body. Chinese people know how to balance their food intake to heal themselves. When the body has too much yin energy, they will use yang food to balance themselves. When the body has too much yang energy, the body needs more yin food for balance. This diet for healing developed, not from scientific study, but from life experiences gathered throughout Chinese history.

In the West, it is popular for nutrition experts to offer advice to patients about a diet they should follow and vitamins and minerals they should take.

Many cancer patients take supplements without telling their doctor.

Information about healing cancer through vitamins and minerals is very confusing and conflicted. Each handbook contains different information and the data from different time periods can vary a great deal. The history of the effectiveness of a vitamin and mineral regimen for healing cancer is short, and each year new scientific data results in new insights.

Unfortunately, conflicting information make the decision about using supplements very confusing and many people abuse supplementation as a strategy for healing. Many patients as well as 'experts' believe that all vitamins and minerals are safe to take, but lately, many reports have emerged about the dangers of overdosing on them. TCM believes that *anything* taken at overdose levels is harmful to the body.

In the West, people very often use a vitamin and mineral regimen in an attempt to heal cancer without any medical knowledge or simply as a precautionary move based on something they heard from someone who read an article or book. Others, such as the Chinese, favor using herbs—they rarely use vitamins. Lately, many in the West have begun to adopt the use of Chinese herbs, though their doctors do not favor this, because many herbs contain harmful chemistry, or poison.

While it is true that Chinese herbs contain poison, patients need to understand that the herbs have two parts. One part, called dispersion type, uses the chemical, or poison, to kill cancer cells or destroy a tumor and it is effective. It is similar to the use of chemo and radiation in the West. Yet, in the west, people may utilize Chinese poison herb therapy while, at the same time, receiving chemo or radiation treatments—this subjects their bodies to increased levels of poison which may cause an overdose situation. In China, chemo and radiation therapy are not commonly used, so when they use these herbs, any harmful side effect is minimal.

Another part of the Chinese herb, called tonification herb, helps build up the Chi. This type of herb usually does not have any side effect, or only a very mild one, and can safely be combined with chemo and radiation therapy. In China, these two types of herb are used together: one to kill the cancer cells, the other one afterward to build up or balance the Chi.

The Chinese herb can be a part of normal diet— many cancer patients cook the herb in their food. Before using Chinese herbs to heal cancer, an herbalist must be consulted in order to determine the appropriate formulation. There are many

Chinese herbs for healing cancer, however, be careful in selecting ones for your own use—utilize a competent herbalist and do not purchase herbs based on advertising claims.

Healing Genetic Cancers

Many experts believe that cancer may be genetic which means it is difficult or impossible to treat, so doctors tell their patients that it is untreatable. In fact, with the Tom Tam Healing System, we treat several genetic diseases such as Down's syndrome, sickle cell anemia, and cerebral palsy.

In order to correct the DNA and heal the genetic disease, the first step is to confirm that the hypothalamus and pituitary glands are functioning normally, because they control growth hormones. This is important because every cell in the body (normal or abnormal) requires growth hormone, and cells become abnormal when these levels are low.

We can find the Ouch point for these endocrine glands on GV22 and BL6 . Of course, blood supply to these areas is important for normal functioning. When the pituitary gland receives normal blood flow, its impulse can be normal.

In 1962, The Nobel Prize in Physiology for Medicine was awarded to Crick, Watson, and Wilkins "for their discoveries concerning the molecular structure of nucleic acids and its significance for information transfer in living material." Their study was of DNA, not of the source of cell function, bioelectricity.

Dr. Knudson believed that cancer is a genetic disease and suggested that multiple "hits" to DNA were necessary to cause cancer. *Proto-oncogenes promote cell growth in a variety of ways. Many can produce hormones, "chemical messengers" between cells that encourage mitosis, the effect of which depends on the signal transduction of the receiving tissue or cells.*

In DNA research, all attention focuses on the "chemical messengers," not the "electrical messengers." Hormones are tangible and can be produced and sold by pharmaceutical companies, so I am not surprised that they concentrate their research attention on hormones, rather than on bioelectricity.

Every year there are news headlines and exciting reports from cancer research institutes about their findings. Yet, do they really work? I contend that the reports are merely a mirage, and the dream to cure cancer will never emerge from this source. Focusing on bioelectricity and its effects on cells may be a better direction for cancer research.

Can Patients Fight Against Cancer?

A patient's first reaction after being diagnosed with cancer is often shock mixed with fear or anger. Many patients ask God or themselves the question, "*Why me?*" This is a natural, instinctual reaction from the human unconscious mind—originating from the hypothalamus which controls the fight or flight response.

Can humans truly fight against cancer? Consider how many people you know of who have survived cancer. Every communication medium seems filled with nothing but bad news about cancer. Those reports repeat this negative message to the point that it becomes embedded in our subconscious and lately has been transformed into fear. The natural reaction to fear is to run away—the "flight" response. Unfortunately, our experience reminds us that we cannot run away from a cancer diagnosis—it is an event we must face head-on.

So how should we deal with the anger? Can we fight the life-altering condition called cancer? Fear and anger cannot help heal cancer, and neither can fight-or-flight responses. According to the fight-flight-or-freeze response, when fight and flight do not help, the only remaining choice is to freeze. Acute stress responses result in a nightmare for the patient and their family, because when the mind is in a 'frozen' state, the patient does not know whom they can trust or depend on, and their thinking is neither clear nor rational. With little forethought or serious consideration, many patients end up trying anything at all in an attempt to eliminate the cancerous condition.

It does not matter what type of cancer a patient is diagnosed with or what stage their cancer is in—the the first problem which must be dealt with is the psychological effect the diagnosis creates. The shock caused by a diagnosis of cancer is a variation of Post-Traumatic Stress Disorder. It is the mind's response to feelings—both perceived and real—of intense helplessness. So in the beginning of treatment, we should pay close attention to releasing the psychological blockage.

In Tong Ren healing, we occasionally see cancer patients cry in our class. This is a healthy emotional or psychological release. After crying, patients feel much better and many of the syndromes are released. When the patient is crying, don't try to comfort them, instead encourage them to cry some more. When humans cry, it changes the endorphins in the brain, which helps release physical or psychological pain. It also may discharge the dysfunction of the sympathetic nervous system and hypothalamus.

In the practice of Tong Ren, many cancer patients are in the terminal stage and have already tried and failed with other healing methods. They come to us to try yet another potential solution. These patients need psychological and spiritual healing in addition to attention to their physical healing. Releasing problems of the mind may help release tension or depression which, in turn, can increase oxygen intake and bioelectricity within their body. This is why most patients feel better after the Tong Ren treatment –they have the ability to take deeper breaths and have increased their oxygen intake.

Are the "Big Three" Effective in Healing Cancer?

There are many methods for healing cancer, but which method should patients choose? It depends on the background of the patient. Each nation has its own way of healing. In the west, the most popular are the "Big Three": surgery, chemotherapy, and radiation therapy.

The main goal of the Big Three is to kill the cancer cells or remove the tumor. Except for a small percentage of inoperable tumors, high-tech surgery is usually effective for eliminating the tumor, and chemotherapy and radiation therapy can destroy tumorous cells. Nevertheless, after removing the tumor and killing any remaining cancer cells, the job is not done. The most difficult job is to prevent new normal cells from mutating into cancerous ones.

The Big Three treatment theory believes that removing the tumor through **surgery** is not enough to eradicate the cancer, and that chemo or radiation must be used to rid the body of any remaining cancer cells. In some cases, chemo or radiation is used first to shrink the tumor, followed by surgery to remove it.

The word cancer is a name for many different diseases and each type of cancer affects the body in its own way. However, all cancers have one thing in common: they are abnormal cells growing out of control. When we treat cancer, removing or killing the cancerous cells is an important part of the process, but the *key* is to stop abnormal cells from growing out of control.

Chemotherapy

Without a doubt, we understand that chemo is a poison—it destroys cancer cells, but destroys healthy cells at the same time. Common side effects of chemotherapy include vomiting, nausea, neuropathy, and a decreased blood count. When white blood cell levels drop (called neutropenia), it can interrupt a patient's chemotherapy schedule and may even be life threatening.

Chemotherapy may put patients at risk for infections and require hospitalization for treatment. During the chemotherapy process, many patients do not die from their cancer, but rather from the side effects of their chemo treatments.

Though we do not deny that chemo can be successful at killing cancer cells, the important question remains: should the patient submit himself to chemotherapy? I cannot answer this question. It is a decision to be made between the individual patient and their doctor, and we, as health practitioners, must respect our patient's will and decision.

Unfortunately, in some cases when a patient does not elect to undergo chemo, they feel that they are missing something in their treatment or that they are not doing enough. They believe that the *only* path toward healing is to kill the cancer. But this is a mainstream medical philosophy.

In the Tom Tam Healing System and Tong Ren healing, we never advise whether or not the cancer patient should use chemo. If the cancer patient is physically strong enough to withstand the treatment or the patient needs it for psychological reasons, why not?

When a patient undergoes chemo, there are usually side effects. Many patients use acupuncture treatments to release some of the uncomfortable effects. Many hospitals have a department where acupuncturists can treat cancer patients. Of course,

Tong Ren healing helps treat the side effects of chemo as well.

Tong Ren practitioners can heal patients over the telephone through a conference call and in live broadcasts of Tong Ren healing through the Internet. In addition, Tong Ren healing offers many classes to help the patient overcome the side effects of chemo.

Radiation

Radiation therapy involves using high doses of radiation to kill cancer cells and stop them from spreading. About 60 percent of cancer patients elect to receive radiation therapy and they report experiencing fewer side effects than from chemo. In some cases, radiation is the only cancer treatment a patient may need.

Radiation may be used to shrink the size of a tumor before surgery, or it may be used after surgery to kill any remaining cancer cells. Sometimes, radiation therapy is given *during* surgery so it goes straight to the cancer without passing through the skin.

During radiation treatment, patients expend a lot of energy to heal, so it is important that they increase their caloric and protein intake to maintain a stable weight during treatment.

Beyond the "Big Three"

After the Big Three are used with success, the next step for the patient is to take a hormone-blocking medication for a few years, or perhaps a target-killing drug for five years. In some cases, patients need to take a mild version of their chemo, in pill form, to continue killing cancer cells or to prevent the cancer cells from growing back.

The Tom Tam Healing System

The Tom Tam Healing System believes that releasing the emotional or psychological problem is the first step in the treatment of cancer. Many cancer patients come to Tong Ren healing classes or receive individual healing with a practitioner, but at the same time still use chemo and/or radiation.

Usually we can use the Tong Ren healing to calm a patient's mind by treating the frontal lobe on GV22, BL6, and Yintang between the eyebrows. Then we bring the Chi downward to the LV3 and K1 points.

After a few minutes, the patient may feel warmth on the face and their palms may get red, which means blood circulation has improved and the Chi is flowing. In some cases, the patient may feel like crying or they may cry uncontrollably during treatment. If a patient wants to cry, encourage them to continue, without fear or judgment.

In Tong Ren healing, when a patient cries, it will benefit their healing result. An emotional release is not required during each Tong Ren treatment, because much of its healing effect will have happened during the first visit. After this first treatment, most patients can calm their own minds and begin to release their stress.

In some terminal cancer cases, we need to pay more attention to the power of the patient's own mind to build confidence in their healing. Through my practice of Tong Ren, many 'terminal' cases have been healed and the patients have gone back to lead normal lives.

The next step is to open the phrenic nerve. We should check LI17 based on palpation if the patient agrees to allow us to touch this point. Through light palpation, we can determine the level of pain the patient is experiencing at this point.

Most cancer patients have a blockage on the left-hand side of LI17. The best technique to open the blockage in the phrenic nerve is to use the Tui Na and Tong Ren combination. After we test the point LI17, based on palpation, we can use the method of Tong Ren with the hammer or other Tong Ren techniques. During the Tong Ren healing, patients may feel warmth on the face or traveling down to the chest or even to the abdomen in the Dantian area.

According to Western medical theory, it is the phrenic nerve function and movement in the diaphragm that cause this area of the Dantian to be active. The Tui Na technique should be applied lightly because many patients experience much pain at LI17 when it is pressed.

The treatment of this area can last five to ten minutes because it is such a sensitive area. After this session, patients may feel a large release of pain and/or emotion as well as the sensation of more oxygen entering the lungs and chest. In addition, some of the pain related to the cancer may be released or even stopped completely.

The next step to treating cancer is to open the blockage on the spinal column where the sympathetic nerve is located. In this step, we must know the patient's official medical diagnosis. Each type of cancer or tumor has a different area, with corresponding blockages, which is responsible for the organ malfunction—there is not just one point that can cover all of the necessary healing.

This is similar to how medical doctors use chemo, knowing that specific chemo drugs are better at treating certain cancers than others. Some people may have multiple tumors or be experiencing the spread of different types of cancer at one time. In this case, we determine where the primary cancer is (based on their medical diagnosis), so we can focus on it first. Later, we can concentrate on the secondary areas containing cancer or tumors.

The last step in treatment is to focus on the "ouch" point. An important Ouch point to focus on is always located where the primary tumor is found as determined by medical scans or examinations, not by an energy diagnosis. The modern approach uses high-tech medical equipment to find the tumor.

Medical scanning equipment includes X-ray, CT scan, MRI scan, and other Western medical tests. Many patients can have pain anywhere in the body as a result of the cancer or for other causative reasons, so the location of pain is not necessarily an indicator of where the cancer exists.

Tong Ren Healing

Tong Ren healing has its own way of healing cancer. One of the techniques is to open the blockage on the phrenic nerve in order to balance the oxygen problem. One thing we have found in Tong Ren practice is that almost all cancer patients have a blockage on the LI17 area.

For most of these, the blockage is on the left-hand side—rarely on the right side. In the Tom Tam Healing System, LI17 is the location on the phrenic nerve which controls the function and movement of the diaphragm.

The point at LI17 is called Tian Ding, which means "Sky Supporter" or "Sky Cup." In Chinese it is also called "Top of Sky." In Traditional Chinese Medicine theory, the head is the sky and the neck is the supporter of the sky. LI17 is located in the neck area 1 cun (inch) directly inferior to LI 18, at the posterior border of the sternocleidomastoid muscle (SCM).

Around LI17 is the superficial cervical artery, external jugular vein, the phrenic nerve, transverse cutaneous nerve of the neck, supraclavicular nerve, and also deep inside is the brachial plexus.

In TCM theory, this point is for healing sore throat, goiter, or tuberculosis cervical lymphadenitis. Its function is for clearing the pharynx and regulating the Chi as well, however, in TCM *practice*, it is rarely used for healing.

In the Tom Tam Healing System, this point is used often—it is a major point for metabolism. Also, it can affect the bronchial nerve, which is formed by the radial nerve, median nerve, and ulna nerve. So when treating shoulder, elbow, and wrist problems, LI17 should be checked.

ST11 affects the phrenic nerve and bronchial nerve as well, and ST12 is where the subclavian arteries pass. When we treat arm, shoulder, or wrist problems, focus should be on ST11 and ST12, which may cause the blockage that affects circulation to the shoulder and hand.

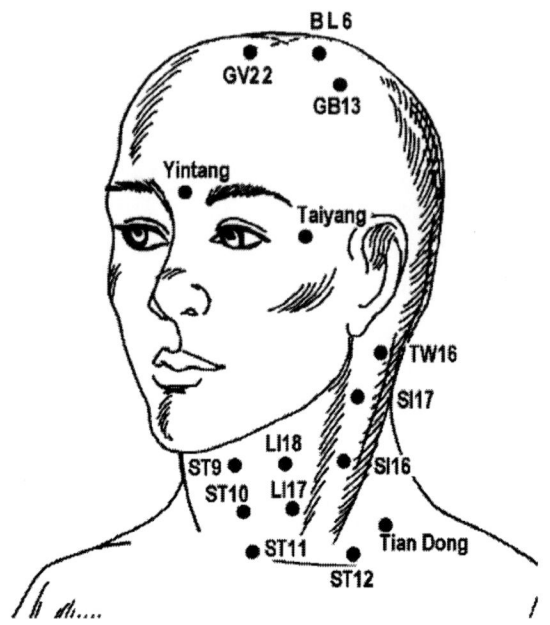

In my practice, I have found that most cancer patients, as well as those struggling with weight issues, have a blockage in LI17. Both cancer and obesity are considered metabolism system imbalances in the Tom Tam Healing System. So, LI17 is a major point for balancing and adjusting the metabolic system.

When we open the blockage in the phrenic nerve, the diaphragm can function normally again. When we open the blockage with LI17, we always check GB 12 as well. GB 12 is on the top of SCM—when the SCM gets tight, it may cause LI17 to become blocked.

Finding Blockages is Key

In the Tom Tam Healing System, there are many methods to stimulate healing within the body, but finding the blockage is more important than which healing technique will be used. Many people get confused and first ask what healing method they should use, but this decision depends upon one's background.

For example, if you are a massage therapist or Tui Na practitioner, you can use your techniques to open the blockage related to the cancer. If you are an acupuncturist, you can use acupuncture needles as a means of stimulation. If you are a physical therapist, you can use the TEN's machine or heat/ice pad. If you are a chiropractor, you can use your method to release the muscular and/or structural problem.

If you do not have any healing knowledge or specific methodology, you can follow the Tong Ren healing chart and use the Tong Ren doll. If you have more people at home, you can use the Tong Ren discing technique or the Tong Ren dowsing method.

Do not needlessly be concerned whether you are working in a correct manner, just use these techniques first, because Tong Ren has no negative side effect or harmful interference with the cancer or other medical conditions. In fact, Tong Ren can help patients build up their energy, which can be damaged by conventional healing methods.

If you want to learn more about Tong Ren healing, you can join a local Tong Ren healing class, or join the live, online healing class that is broadcast on a regular basis. Many people worldwide learn how to use our technique by simply watching the online class.

Many diseases cannot be treated with only the Eastern or Western medical system and I believe that this is the reason more diseases cannot be treated successfully. We need to combine several healing philosophies into a new effective way of healing.

If experts could put aside stubborn biases from their own concepts and standard education, then many so-called incurable and difficult diseases can be treated easily. The Tom Tam Healing System combines Western and Eastern medical theories and has healed many difficult, 'incurable', and rare diseases.

Healing Specific Cancers

Pancreatic Cancer

Problems of the pancreas are difficult to treat, as evidenced by diabetes, hypoglycemia, pancreatitis, and the worst pancreatic disease, cancer. The American Cancer Society estimates that there were 42,470 new cases of pancreatic cancer and 35,240 deaths from pancreatic cancer in America during 2009. Pancreatic cancer is the tenth most common cancer in men and women, and the fourth leading cause of cancer death in men and women.

Pancreatic cancer is difficult to detect, and is often not diagnosed until after it has spread to other parts of the body. The pancreatic cancer survival rate is low, less than five percent of Americans with pancreatic cancer survive five years past diagnosis.

The exact causes of pancreatic cancer are still unknown according to medical studies, but researchers are aware of certain high risk factors: age, gender, race, cigarette smoking, diet, diabetes, environment, and family history.

Scientists have discovered that cancer cells develop from damaged DNA. Under normal circumstances, when DNA becomes damaged, the body is able to repair it, but in the case of cancer cells, the damaged DNA is not repaired.

How can DNA become damaged? Scientists believe that it is damaged by exposure to harmful environmental elements. To keep DNA functioning normally, and to heal any cancer, including pancreatic cancer, we need to study both biochemical and bioelectrical effects on DNA. Unfortunately, scientists are interested in cell structure, external factors, and biochemical effects, and ignore internal factors such as nerves and bioelectricity, yet different levels of bioelectricity in the body will cause different functions in the DNA.

The pancreas is a glandular organ located behind the stomach which extends across the abdomen horizontally, and is surrounded by the small intestine, liver, and spleen. It is about six inches long and less than two inches wide, including three parts: the head, the body, and the tail. Its head is on the right side of the abdomen, in an area behind the stomach joining with the first part of the small intestine; the body is located behind the stomach; and the tail is on the left side of the abdomen next to the spleen.

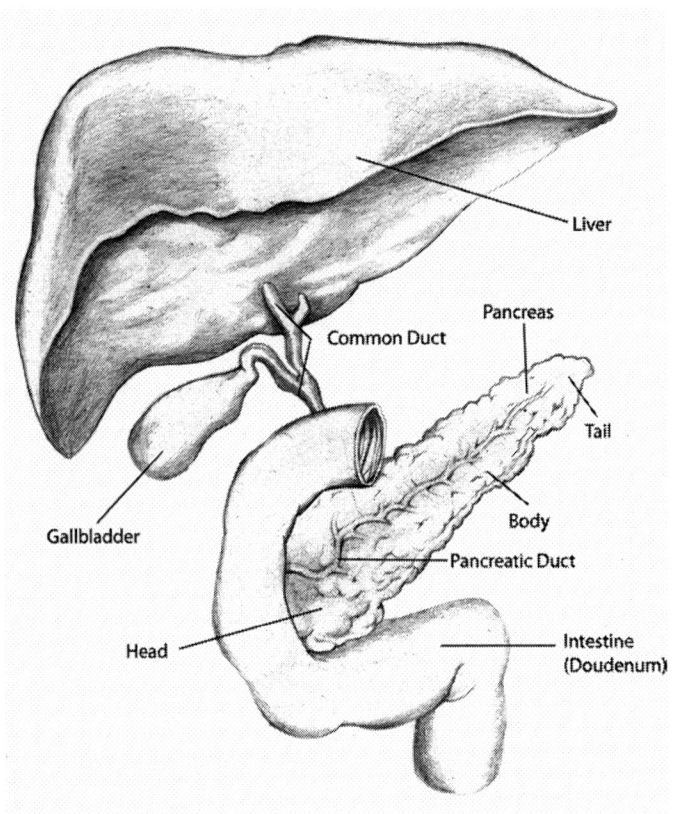

Due to the pancreas' location, determining a healing strategy can be confusing. According to the Tom Tam Healing System, the blockage relating to the function of the pancreas is located at the right side of T8. However, in practice we find the right side of both T7 and T8 often have an Ouch point. Sometimes we can find the blockage on the left side of T7 and T8. Therefore, when healing any pancreatic problem, we need to focus on both sides on the spinal column to be certain nothing is missed.

The pancreas contains two different types of glands: exocrine and endocrine. The pancreatic function is controlled from the pituitary gland in the brain (where growth hormone is produced). When we treat pancreatic disease, we need to focus on GV22 and BL6, which are located in the frontal lobe area and control hormone function.

In terms of physiology, any cell's growth depends on growth hormone. If the growth hormone cannot send an impulse to the pancreas, it can cause the cell to grow out of control and become abnormal.

More than 95 percent of the cells in the pancreas are found in the exocrine glands and ducts. These glands make pancreatic "juice" which contains enzymes. It is released into the intestines to help digest fats, proteins, and carbohydrates from food. When enzymes are low, some food may pass through the intestines without being absorbed—this is the reason pancreatic cancer causes weight loss.

The pancreatic enzymes are released into small ducts which merge together to form larger ducts which carry the pancreatic juice to the small intestine for absorption. Many Ton Ren patients gain weight during their treatment because the pancreas resumes production of its juice and absorption of food.

Only a small percentage of pancreatic cells are endocrine cells, and these are arranged in small clusters called Islets of Langerhans. These islets release two important hormones directly into the blood: insulin and glucagon. Insulin reduces the amount of sugar in the blood, while glucagon increases it. Diabetes results from a defect in insulin production.

Chronic pancreatitis is considered long-term inflammation of the pancreas. Logically, it should be linked with an increased risk of pancreatic cancer, but studies of most patients with pancreatitis reveal they never develop this cancer. This puzzles the scientist, however, the explanation is easy when viewed through the Tom Tam Healing System: pancreatitis is not a pancreas problem, but rather an immune system problem.

According to Western medical study, pancreatic cancer is more common in people with Type 2 Diabetes, typically with adulthood onset, and often those patients who are overweight. So how can Type 2 Diabetes increase the risk of pancreatic cancer? Because a cell's growth is a metabolic function and Type 2 Diabetes is a metabolic problem. Type 1 Diabetes is an auto-immune system problem with no link to pancreatic cancer, which means that the immune system is *not* the main cause of this cancer. Yet, Western doctors focus, erroneously, on the immune system rather the metabolic system.

Healing Cancer with the Nervous System

The Tom Tam Healing System has a high rate of success with treating pancreatic cancer. The major technique is to open the blockage on the left-hand side of the phrenic nerve at LI17 (In our practice, only a small percentage of patients have a blockage on the right-hand side at this point). When we lightly press LI17, the cancer patient will feel pain, so in the early stages of treatment Tui Na massage should be used lightly to open this blockage.

If possible, the patient's family, or even the patient himself, can do this style of massage daily. Usually using Tui Na and Tong Ren in combination brings a good result to open this blockage. We also need to check the point of ST11 for sensitivity or pain also located on the pathway of the phrenic nerve.

As for people with Type 1 Diabetes, it is still unclear whether they have a higher-than-average risk of developing pancreatic cancer. To decrease the occurrence of pancreatic cancer, diabetes must be stopped, but to date, modern medicine can only *control* diabetes to a degree, not *heal* it.

In Tong Ren healing, diabetes is prevented by keeping T7 and T8 on the right side open. When healing the diabetic patient, one can use the laser beam on ST21 on the doll, and can also hammer T7 and T8 on the right side. This technique applies to the treatment of pancreatic cancer as well.

Neither of these techniques, by themselves, have the power to treat pancreatic cancer as effectively as Tom Tam's discing technique. Why is the discing technique more effective than other Tong Ren healing techniques? At this point we cannot give a definitive explanation, so we simply observe the results in practice.

The discing technique (which is a form of energy healing) is simple and will work for anyone willing to do it—it requires no special training. Its healing power is formed by a group's mind, a combination of the collective consciousness and collective unconsciousness.

Before using the discing technique for treating pancreatic cancer, we should check the patient's Ouch point in the abdomen at ST21, both right and left sides. Most patients will feel pain or discomfort in this area. Also we can check ST25, located four fingers' width beside the navel. When we find the Ouch point in the abdomen, we put the disk on the top of the Ouch point, or allow the patient to put it where they feel most discomfort.

After using the discing technique for five minutes, compare the Ouch point with the same palpatory test. In most cases, pain decreases and the Ouch point may even disappear. The next step in discing is to treat the back on the T7 and T8 area. Usually, the Ouch point is found on the right side of the spine, but in some cases may be on the left. Most pancreatic cancer patients have a large blockage in this area, and many of them have a curvature of the spinal column, mainly bending to the right side of the body.

To enhance the healing effect, we can use Tui Na massage in conjunction with acupuncture for correcting the blockage. In some cases, Tong Ren healing alone is not powerful enough to open the blockage in the spinal area because the tissue in this area is too tight.

Because the pancreas is related to hormonal problems, and the pituitary gland controls hormones, we focus on the BL6 and GV22 area to charge the pituitary. After discing on T7 and T8, we place the disc for a few minutes on GV22 (which also covers BL6).

The circulation of the pituitary is through the vertebral artery, so we may find a blockage in the TW16 and TW17 area as well. To open the vertebral artery's blockage of energy, we can put a small disk in the Tian Dong, SI16, TW16 and TW17. Most pancreatic cancer patients feel better after the discing technique and some of their symptoms may be released.

In the Tom Tam Healing System, the sympathetic nerve runs down the back of the body and the parasympathetic nerve runs from the neck area down the kidney meridian on the front of the body. With Tong Ren healing, we can use the hammer technique to open the vagus nerve in the neck area, then follow the kidney meridian from K27 (located under the collarbone) down to ST21 on both sides of the torso.

With the laser technique, we can focus the laser beam on ST21 for a daily treatment. Patients with a blood sugar imbalance should monitor their blood sugar levels, since after a Tong Ren healing blood sugar levels may be more balanced. If so, patients should seek medical advice to adjust their medications.

There are many different types of pancreatic cancer, which medical experts may explain in detail to their patients. Accordingly, different chemotherapies are prescribed for different types of cancer. However, in Tong Ren healing, no matter what form of pancreatic cancer, the treatment is basically the same.

For healing purposes, we focus on the primary cancer in the pancreas, but when pancreatic cancer cells are carried through the bloodstream to affect the liver, lungs, bone, or other organs, it is called metastatic pancreatic cancer. When this happens, we refer to the cancer in the affected organ(s) as secondary and treat those organs as Ouch points.

To heal the pancreas we need to correct diet. Some diet studies have found a link between pancreatic cancer and diets high in fat, which include a large amount of red meat, pork, and processed meat, such as sausage and bacon. Some diet studies have found that diets high in fruits and vegetables may help reduce the risk of pancreatic cancer.

The Tom Tam Healing System stresses the importance of eliminating soda with artificial sweeteners from the diet. Many Americans still favor diet drinks and believe that sugar substitutes are healthy. The calories in the soda are not the culprits, but the chemicals in the drink and the sugar substitute—they can destroy the pancreas and liver.

During Tong Ren healing sessions, I always advise patients to stop ingesting these junk foods. I also discourage patients with pancreatic problems from taking supplements. In America, people take supplements as a daily routine. In fact, most people take vitamins or supplements "just in case" instead of determining whether they have a true deficiency that requires treatment. I recommend supplements only for a diagnosed deficiency, never for psychological reasons.

Some researchers believe that excess stomach acid may increase the risk of pancreatic cancer. The stomach is located in the same part of the abdomen as the pancreas (which in TCM is called the middle warmer). The nerve for the stomach is next to the pancreas, so when one of these organs becomes blocked, it may affect the other.

Another factor which may increase the risk of developing pancreatic cancer is an infection of the stomach caused from ulcerative bacteria, known as helicobacter pylori. When healing pancreatic cancer, we must also consider the stomach function. Many pancreatic cancer patients use chemotherapy or radiation, which may destroy the stomach's function, so to build up stomach energy, we can use the laser beam on the middle warmer and lower warmer points, at CV12 and CV4, respectively.

Some types of pancreatic cancer are considered hereditary and approximately 10 percent of cases may be related to inherited DNA mutations. These changes often increase the risk for certain other cancers as well. Tong Ren healing approaches the genetic problem by relating any cell mutations to the growth hormone.

Since growth hormone is produced from the pituitary gland, when that gland is out of balance, it may cause any of the so-called 'genetic' diseases. When using Tong Ren healing for an inherited DNA mutation, focus the energy on the BL6 and GV22.

Most pancreatic cancer patients use chemotherapy for their treatment, and a high percentage of them submit to a clinical drug trial and place their hope in the new drug, even though healing rates with drugs is still very low.

In my observations over the last ten years, pancreatic cancer patients appear to drain more energy when undergoing chemotherapy than any other type of cancer patient. Thus the pancreatic cancer patient should carefully weigh the benefits of chemo.

When treating pancreatic cancer patients, we should include healing for psychological problems as well. For the most part, when patients hear that they have an 'incurable' disease, it may cause them to lose confidence and give up the fight for healing. The best way to build up patients' confidence is to accompany them to a Tong Ren healing class, so they can talk to other cancer patients about their experience with Tong Ren therapy.

Breast Cancer

In America, breast cancer is second only to lung cancer as the leading cause of cancer deaths among women, and it is the leading cause of cancer death for women ages forty to fifty-five. Breast cancer might be the most feared disease by women because it is so common yet its causes remain mostly unknown. In fact, only heart disease is more common and dangerous than breast cancer. Even though heart disease is the number-one killer in America, women pay more attention to their breasts and hair than to their hearts, because they are symbols of beauty and sexuality for women. Therefore, breast cancer can affect a woman's body image and self-esteem.

The risk of developing breast cancer increases greatly after age forty with about 80 percent of invasive breast cancers turning up in women over fifty—and the older a woman gets, the greater the risk. So, in the West, experts believe it is a good idea for women to continue with mammograms, clinical exams, and breast self-exams well into their seventies and eighties.

Since 1960, the rate of breast cancer in America has jumped from one in fourteen women to one in eight. Around 200,000 new cases of invasive breast cancer are diagnosed in women each year and about 40,000 women a year die from breast cancer. Right now, the United States has more than 2.5 million breast cancer survivors either in treatment, or having completed treatment.

Why has the rate of breast cancer increased and not decreased? Considering the rapid developments in modern medicine and improvements in the environment since the sixties, this is a confusing statistic. The more questions we ask, the more confusing the conversation gets. Also, breast cancer doesn't only occur in women—it is also being recognized in men, and the breast cancer rate for men has jumped as well (and I use the same technique for healing both genders).

Types of Breast Cancer

As we know, cancer is caused by normal cells exhibiting abnormal function, such as a high rate of mutation and excessive growth—and these are characterized as a metabolism problem. At the same time, there is a rare form of breast cancer related to the immune system, called Inflammatory Breast Cancer (IBC).

IBC may occur with inflammation, skin redness, and breast pain, however, this does not mean that IBC symptoms are caused by infection or injury. The symptoms of IBC are caused by cancer cells blocking lymph vessels in the skin. IBC tends to occur in younger women, and African American women appear to be at higher risk than Caucasians.

Symptoms of IBC can develop very quickly and more aggressively than the more common types of breast cancer. When IBC is diagnosed, it is generally at least stage IIIB (locally advanced) and may be stage IV (metastatic) if it has spread to distant parts of the body. Studies have shown that over the past couple of decades, IBC has become more common, while other forms of locally advanced breast cancer have become less common—researchers are still not sure why.

Other breast cancers include Invasive Ductal Carcinoma (IDC Breast Cancer), Invasive Lobular Carcinoma (ILC Breast Cancer), and Lobular carcinoma in situ (LCIS), which means that there are cell changes inside the breast lobes. (LCIS is not cancer, and though most women with LCIS will not get breast cancer, those with LCIS can be at an increased risk of breast cancer in the future.)

Treating Breast Cancer

IBC is often more difficult to treat successfully than other types of breast cancer. In fact, in the case of any diagnosis relating to the immune system, Western medicine does not have a good track record for healing.

However, the use of the Tom Tam Healing System can often bring good results in healing immune system problems through the use of stimulation to the nerves at T1, T2, and T3, which causes an increase in immune system function. Treatment through the Tom Tam Healing System is the same for all types of breast cancer since the blockages are the same.

Western medicine believes that the best method for successfully treating breast cancer is early detection—of course, any cancer, if found early enough, is easier to treat. When breast cancer is treated in the early stages, the five-year survival rate is around 95 percent, while in cases of Stage 4, the five-year survival rate is low, at about 20 percent.

Early detection theory keeps changing, as reported through the media, making it confusing for women and experts alike. The medical establishment advises monthly self breast exams and annual clinical breast exams for women age 20 and older, combined with annual mammograms for women ages forty and older, as these are considered the best methods for early detection.

Some health insurance companies require their customers to have annual mammograms. Doctors believe that an annual mammogram for women aged fifty and older would reduce the death rate by 30 percent. Yet, in these modern times, many women still object to mammograms for a variety of reasons.

Clearly, a mammogram does not prevent breast cancer—it is simply a means of detecting breast tumors and more than 20 percent of mammograms miss detecting breast cancer. In addition, many experts believe that mammograms can *cause* breast and other forms of cancer, adding to the confusion.

In the Tom Tam Healing System, the concepts are much simpler. Monthly, a woman can have anyone (no need for an expert) check the area of the back lateral to T4, LI17, and BL9. Some women enjoy the services of a massage therapist once a month. If so, they can ask their therapist to work on the T4 area for five to ten minutes, and also on LI17, which is located on the neck.

I deeply believe that the T4 and LI17 blockages are the root cause of breast cancer, but one need not panic if they find blockages at those locations—it does not mean that breast cancer is present; however, with a diagnosed case of breast cancer, the major blockage will be at T4, on the same side of the body which has the cancer.

Women who detect their breast cancer early can choose from a variety of treatment choices. In addition to a mastectomy, women who meet certain criteria may have the option of breast conservation therapy (BCT).

BCT involves removal of just the area of cancerous tissue with follow-up radiation therapy. When there are many areas of cancer in the breast, or the tumor is almost as large as the breast itself, a mastectomy is a better choice. For many women, it is difficult to imagine that less surgery is equal in value to more surgery.

For some women, though, BCT may not be cosmetically desirable, in 20 years of comparative studies between BCT and mastectomy, the survival rates are the same.

I don't have to remind you that medical studies are confusing. Reports advise that a low-fat, high-fiber diet along with regular exercise cannot guarantee complete protection against breast cancer but may reduce the risk of developing it. Most studies have not found smoking to be a *cause* of breast cancer, but many have found a *link* between the two, and some research indicates that smoking can hinder a woman's chances of surviving the disease after being diagnosed.

There is no approved treatment that can eliminate a woman's risk of breast cancer. However, a drug called Tamoxifen has been approved by the FDA for use by high-risk women to decrease their risk of developing the disease. It is also often taken by women after receiving treatment for breast cancer.

Tamoxifen has been shown to significantly reduce the risk of breast cancer by around 45 percent. Like all drugs, though, it has side effects. It may cause uterine cancer and blood clotting, and may have other side effects which are still unknown. It will be years before we know the percentage of women taking this drug who remain disease-free.

Raloxifene is a drug similar to Tamoxifen, but it acts more selectively in helping to decrease the risk of breast cancer. It has not been shown to cause potentially cancerous changes in the lining of the uterus, however, it does carry the same risk of blood clotting. Whether or not to take a drug like Tamoxifen or Raloxifene must be made on a case-by-case basis. It reduces one's risk of cancer but raises other risks and side effects. Many breast cancer patients take these types of medicine more for psychological benefits than physical ones.

In my practice, all women who have breast cancer or cysts have one thing in common: a blockage in the T4 and LI17 areas. Most have a blockage on the same side as the cancer. In the T4 area, we can see puffing or skin marks such as a mole, rash, or red petechiae. In my healing philosophy, T4 is a Chi passageway to the breast and controls sweat glands, hair follicles, and skin problems including skin cancer, melanomas, and psoriasis. LI17 is the phrenic nerve, which may increase the oxygen needed to correct cell mutation.

My healing way is intended to reduce the risk of breast cancer and to keep T4 and LI17 open. The easiest and most effective way is to use the Tui Na massage technique. In addition, exercises such as Chi Gong, Tai Chi, Yoga, or any type of stretching in the T4 area is valuable. Even the use of a massage machine on that area can help to open a blockage.

The major causes of T4 and LI17 blockages are poor posture when typing, doing computer work, holding the telephone, reading, carrying, or even lifting weights. Accidents or traumas, as in the case of a car accident, can also cause a T4 blockage to develop over time.

During a Tong Ren treatment, the patient will feel warmth on the face first, and then the warmth will go down the neck into the shoulders and pass into the breast area. Sometimes the patient may feel a tingling sensation instead while others report feeling only relaxation. In fact, a relaxed feeling is a sign of healing. When the body is relaxed, bioelectricity can flow easily.

When practicing Tong Ren and Chi Gong to treat breast cancer, sometimes what seems like a miracle may occur: after five to ten minutes, the tumor may become significantly smaller and softer. The patient can monitor these changes herself if the tumor can be touched or held during treatment.

As it is held, the patient should remember the size and tension of the tumor so she can detect changes. Occasionally, the tumor may completely disappear. This is not a staged magician's performance; it is a healing phenomenon of the practice of Chi Gong.

Many people will wonder how a tumor can shrink or disappear during such a short time. However, this sometimes also happens in medical studies. When a tumor has been passed over with positive bioelectricity, we have seen the tumor shrink or disappear. When the tumor gets smaller or disappears, it does not mean the cancer is gone, so a doctor still must be consulted to determine the next step—to check for cancer cells and tumors is their job, not ours.

During a Tong Ren or Chi Gong treatment, not only can a tumor shrink but lymph nodes can shrink as well. In some cases where the breast was swollen, the swelling may disappear as well as the tumor. Many times in the early stages of breast cancer, during a Tong Ren treatment, the tumor may disappear before surgery is performed. If the tumor disappears, we must explain the theory behind it, but do not mislead the patient into any form of superstition or mystery—we work with concepts founded in science, not religion.

When a tumor disappears, a CAT scan will show nothing. The doctor will often not believe what has happened and still suggest surgery and radiation—and the patient is usually willing to accept this. We cannot give any opinion to a patient in this case because, psychologically, they believe that radiation after surgery is the best way to work towards prevention.

Healing Cancer with the Nervous System

It is natural for a breast cancer patient to feel depressed and about 25 percent of patients will have depression when taking medication. Tong Ren has shown good results in relieving depression. We can use the right side of GB13 or C2 and T5. If the symptoms are severe and long-lasting, we should aim the Tong Ren laser on the frontal lobe of the Tong Ren doll to alleviate the depression.

Another confusing issue within current medical studies is why black women have a lower breast cancer rate than white women. My theory is logical and easy to understand. The darker the skin color, the more melanin pigment is in the body.

According to anatomy and physiology, melanin (which is produced from the pituitary gland's anterior lobe) protects the skin. The pituitary gland controls growth, prolactin, and adrenocorticotropic hormones, which synthesize melanin's melanocyte-stimulating hormone. Darker skin will absorb more sunlight, making it necessary for the body to radiate more heat.

The human body releases heat through a function of the sweat glands. We know that darker colors absorb more heat from sunlight than lighter ones, so dark-skinned people need more active sweat glands to release the heat than light-skinned people do—and we observe that black women do have more enriched sweat glands and mammary glands than white women.

The Tom Tam Healing System postulates that blockages relating to breast cancer can also be found in the chest, on the kidney meridian. Usually we can find the Ouch point on K24 or K23.

The breast organ is controlled by the pituitary gland but it doesn't matter if the bio-signal comes from the pituitary gland or the hypothalamus, because the reflex points for both are BL6 and GV22. So when we treat any of the endocrine cancers or tumors, we should pay attention to those two points. It is a new theory that we should use the pituitary gland point for breast cancer, but it is not strange to use this point if we believe that the mammary gland is connected to the pituitary gland.

Colon Cancer

When first detected, cancer in the colon is called colon cancer, and cancer in the rectum is called rectal cancer. As with other cancers, medical science does not understand the cause. Colon cancer is one of the most common cancers in America. About 50,000 people die from it each year. About one in 20 Americans will get colorectal cancer in his or her lifetime.

For early detection, doctors suggest people start having rectal examinations at age 40. Regular screening for blood in the stool should be done for everyone aged 50 and older; this exam may establish early detection in those with risk factors.

Many believe that colon cancer results from diet, because the colon, along with the rectum, is a part of the digestive system. Some experts also believe that family history may relate with the possible risk of colon cancer, and some believe that a personal history of inflammatory bowel disease such as Crohn's, colitis, or adenomatous polyps can prove to be responsible for the development of colon cancer.

Others believe that smoking or drinking alcohol can cause colon cancer. The other concern has to do with age, as most patients with colorectal cancer are over age 50. In this age bracket, many people may develop polyps (which are a natural and common occurrence) and some types may increase a person's risk of developing colorectal cancer.

Through research, doctors have found that there is a rare inherited condition called familial polyposis, which can cause hundreds of polyps to form in the colon and rectum and results in greater risk of getting colorectal cancer.

Other possible causes are: ulcerative colitis, a condition in which the lining of the colon becomes inflamed; medical history, such as women who have had cancer of the ovary, uterus, or breast; and someone having had colorectal cancer once before then developing the disease a second time. A doctor may also have concern if there is a family history of the cancer, for chances increase even more in those cases.

The colon and rectum form the large intestine, or large bowel. The colon is a long muscular tube about six feet long, and the rectum, which is about eight to ten inches long, is the last part of large intestine.

The autonomic nervous system controls the movement of the large intestine, which is where water, electrolytes, and vitamin K from food as well as waste are stored. And because the large intestine is a long tube, the complex branch of nerves can easily develop blockages.

When the rectum is filled with waste products, the autonomic nerves should cause the rectum to become active and allow the waste to pass from the body; if the autonomic nerve is blocked, the bowel will not move properly.

The autonomic nervous system is divided into the sympathetic and parasympathetic systems: one controls the increase of organ movement and the other controls the decrease of organ movement.

Early Detection and Preventative Measures are Important

Medical research shows that colorectal cancer develops gradually from benign polyps, so early detection and removal of polyps is an important way to reduce risk and prevent this cancer. Most studies in America look for external factors which can cause colorectal cancer, such as smoking and alcohol use, use of dietary supplements, aspirin, or similar medicines, and getting into a regular physical exercise program.

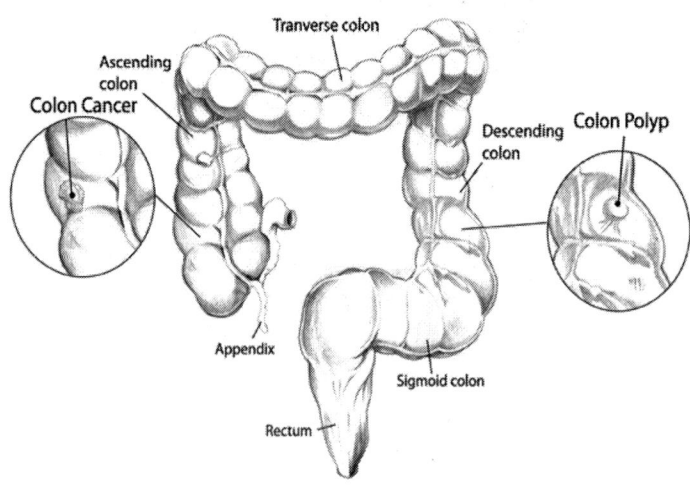

Some experts suggest that a diet low in fat and calories and high in fiber can help prevent colorectal cancer. In fact, this type of preventative measure is indicated not only for colorectal cancer but for all cancers. Western medicine states that following cancer-preventative methods can decrease risk by a small percentage, however, none is a true preventative because Western medicine, along with modern science, still has not discovered the cause of cancer.

How are polyps formed and how should colitis or constipation be treated? Experts have not yet found an effective way to treat this because they focus on diet and exercise only. If we cannot treat colitis and effectively stop the growth of polyps, how can we prevent colon cancer?

In my practice, this problem is easily treated and the success rate is high. I believe that digestive problems are caused by blockages in the autonomic nervous system that controls intestinal functions, therefore, my treatment for a digestive disorder focuses on the blockage, not on diet.

Testing for Colon Cancer

Everyone agrees that the best preventative measure for colon cancer is early detection, including Traditional Chinese Medicine which believes in the concept of "healing the disease before it occurs." A popular and frequently used test for detection is the FOBT (fecal occult blood test), used to check for hidden blood in the stool, because some cancers or polyps can bleed.

A sigmoidoscopy is an examination of the rectum and sigmoid colon done with a sigmoidoscope.

Colonoscopy is an examination of the rectum and entire colon done with a colonoscope. An x-ray used to check the colon and rectum is called the DCBE (double-contrast barium enema). The DRE (digital rectal exam) is an exam in which the doctor inserts a lubricated and gloved finger into the rectum to feel for abnormal areas. No matter what type of exam is used, it is only a test to find an intestinal problem. There are still no proven techniques that can completely *prevent* colorectal cancer.

Symptoms which will lead a doctor to advise a colorectal exam include diarrhea, constipation, blood in the stool, narrower-shaped stools than usual, abdominal discomfort, weight loss for unknown reasons, vomiting, and fatigue. After a doctor has diagnosed colon cancer, he needs to determine the stage of the cancer, because different stages have different treatments. If the cancer cells have spread to other parts of the body, additional tests will be needed.

Stages of Cancer

The earliest stage is Stage 0. Stage 0 is when the cancer cells are found in the innermost lining of the colon or rectum only. Stage I is still considered 'early' detection and means that the cancer involves more of the inner wall of the colon or rectum. In the early stages, the five-year survival rate is as high as 95 percent. In Stage II, the cancer has spread from the inside to the outside of the intestine, but not yet into the lymph nodes.

In Stage III, the cancer has spread to nearby lymph nodes but not other organs. If the cancer has spread to the lymph nodes, the five-year survival rate drops to 50 percent. In Stage IV, the cancer has spread to other organs such as the liver or lung. This is a 'late' stage for which the five-year survival rate is less than 10 percent. When cancer returns after a doctor's medical treatment, it is called recurrent cancer, and may reoccur in the colon, in the rectum, or in another part of the body. With colon cancer, the recurrent cancer rate is high.

Treatment of Colorectal Cancer

After the stage of the cancer has been determined, the doctor plans its treatment. Generally, no matter what the stage is, the first method considered is surgery. Psychologically, everyone believes if the cancerous part of the intestine is removed, the cancer will be gone. It sounds logical; doctors can successfully remove tumors from anywhere in the intestine, but they *cannot* remove the blockage which may have *caused* the cancer. The surgery used is dependent upon the size of the tumor, the involvement of regional lymph nodes, how far the cancer has spread, and the individual case. The size of the tumor has little influence on prognosis or the follow-up method of treatment.

After surgery, a doctor may use chemotherapy, which is an adjuvant therapy used to kill any remaining cancer cells. Chemo is usually begun about one month after surgery and continues for six to twelve months and may be in IV form or pill form.

With rectal cancer, doctors may use radiation therapy *before* surgery to kill the cancer cells and shrink the tumor—this can make the tumor easier to remove. Sometimes doctors may use radiation to destroy any cancer cells that remain in the treated area *after* surgery. Doctors believe that radiation therapy (which may be internal and/or external) relieves symptoms associated with colorectal cancer. The most popular form of radiation used to stop cancer cells from proliferating is x-rays or gamma rays.

When Tong Ren and Tui Na therapy are combined with a doctor's treatment, the recurrence rate drops significantly. In a Tong Ren treatment, we first find and open the intestinal blockage, no matter what stage the patient is in. If the cancer cells have spread to other organs, we follow the Spinal Chart to find out where the secondary blockage is located. During Tong Ren healing, some patients' tumors come out of the body during a bowel movement—don't be surprised if this happens.

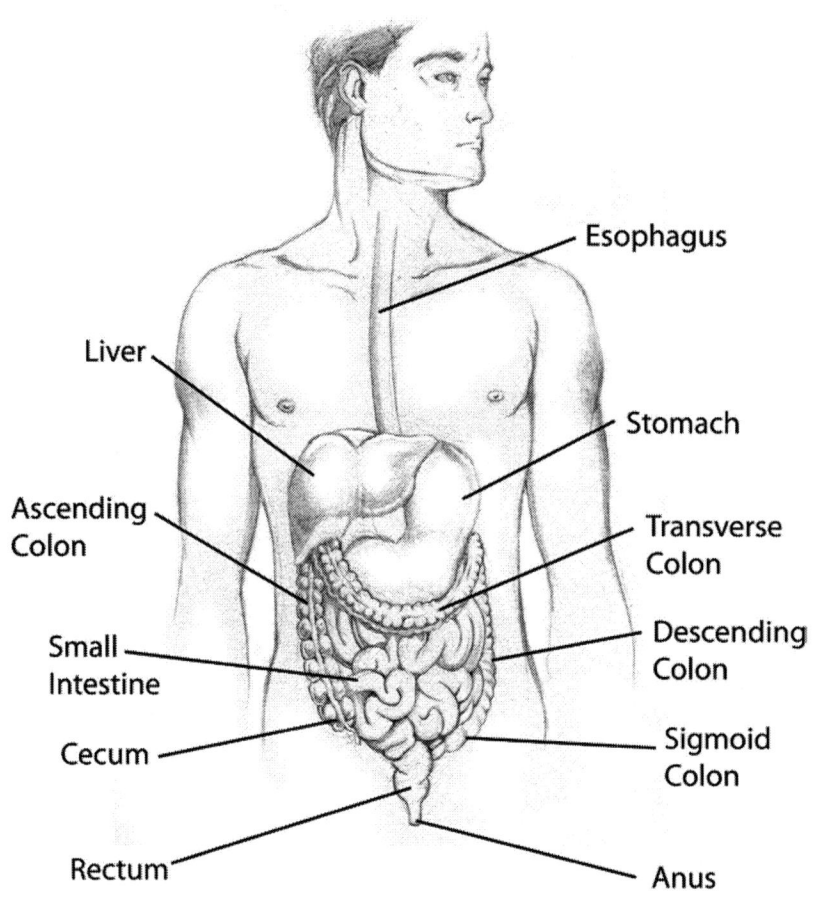

Biological therapies and clinical trials are also available for colorectal cancer patients. The theory behind biological therapy is to boost the immune system so the body will naturally kill the cancer cells. With Tog Ren therapy, the immune system can be improved without side effects.

Western treatment for colorectal cancer will have side effects. Often a patient misunderstands or is misled into thinking that biological therapy has no side effects, or that it is a 'new' cure. I never believe any new development comes with few or no side effects—if a drug's purpose is to kill cells, it *will* have harmful side effects.

For patients receiving the "Big-Three", Tong Ren or acupuncture and energy-healing are recommended. When these treatments are used in combination, a patient will heal much more quickly.

After treatment, a doctor will want to watch for any possible developments of the disease and many tests, including the carcinoembryonic antigen (CEA) blood test, will be required. Many patients pay too much attention to the CEA test. When the CEA number drops down, the patient will become very excited; if it goes up, they will become very disappointed, perhaps even depressed.

We cannot deny the CEA test results, but don't be overly influenced by them. Researchers have found that this test has missed many recurrences and also resulted in false positives, requiring additional expensive tests, and even surgery in some cases, to rule out cancer. I believe that a patient's instinctive feeling is more important than the CEA test. It is my understanding that sometimes when the CEA rises, it means the body is becoming more active in cleansing toxins out of the bowel.

Lung Cancer

Lung cancer is the leading cause of cancer deaths among both men and women. Currently, more women are dying each year of lung cancer than of breast cancer. The one-year survival rate for lung cancer patients is about 40 percent and the five-year survival rate is about 14 percent.

Symptoms may include repeated problems with pneumonia or bronchitis, swelling of the neck and face, fatigue, a low-grade fever, weight loss, and loss of appetite. It is important to check with a medical doctor in order to detect cancer in its early stages—they should be consulted for symptoms that include constant chest pain, a persistent cough that worsens over time, or a cough with bloody phlegm, shortness of breath, wheezing, or hoarseness. Because cancer rates are high, people fear getting cancer, so some lung symptoms may be psychosomatic.

Types of Lung Cancer

There are two major types of cancer that begin in the lungs: divided, non-small-cell lung cancer and small-cell lung cancer. The type diagnosed depends on what the cells look like when examined under a microscope. Each type grows and spreads in different ways, and is treated differently by doctors. About 75 percent of lung cancers are of the non-small-cell variety, and the remaining cases are classified as small-cell lung cancers.

There are three main types of non-small cell lung cancers: squamous cell carcinoma (also called epidermoid carcinoma), adenocarcinoma, and large cell carcinoma. Small-cell lung cancer is sometimes called oat cell cancer. This type of lung cancer is less common than, and different from, the non-small-cell lung cancer in that it grows faster and spreads more easily to other organs.

Tumors in the lung can be benign or malignant. Benign tumors are not cancerous and its cells do not spread to other parts of the body. Most importantly, benign tumors are seldom life-threatening. In most cases, a benign tumor can be removed and, when done, does not come back.

Malignant tumors, on the other hand, are cancerous and can threaten life. The cancerous cells in malignant tumors are abnormal and divide without control or order. These cancer cells can invade and destroy the tissue around them, and they can also break away from a tumor and enter the bloodstream or lymphatic system.

Lung Anatomy and Function

The lungs—which are a pair of sponge-like, cone-shaped organs—are part of the respiratory system located in the thoracic cavity. The right lung has three sections called lobes—it is a little larger in size than the left lung, which has two lobes.

When we inhale, the lungs take in oxygen, which our cells need to live and carry out their normal functions. When we exhale, the lungs get rid of carbon dioxide, which is a waste product of the body's cells. Neither of the lungs moves on its own, instead all lung movement—inhalation and exhalation—comes from, and is controlled by, the movement of the diaphragm.

Diagnosing Lung Cancer

A Tong Ren therapist never diagnoses cancer—that is a doctor's responsibility. However, in some cases it is difficult to detect lung cancer in its early stage because the disease spreads quickly and symptoms often do not appear until the disease is advanced. Only 15 percent of lung cancers are found before the cells have spread to lymph nodes or other organs.

To diagnose lung cancer, doctors will perform a physical exam, take a chest x-ray, and possibly order other tests. If lung cancer is suspected, sputum cytology is a simple test that can be useful in detection. Despite the use of these tests, a biopsy is the only way to *definitively prove* a diagnosis for the presence of lung cancer. Relatively easy techniques for biopsy are bronchoscopes, needle aspiration, and thoracentesis. Some biopsies require major surgery called thoracotomy, which is the opening of the chest in order to make a diagnosis.

Causes of Lung Cancer

When someone you know is diagnosed with lung cancer, you may be shocked at first, assuming that it must have been caused by smoking. In fact, a person may never smoke and still get lung cancer. Then, logically, the complaint turns to secondhand smoke (involuntary or passive smoking). If the patient's home and workplace are smoke-free, then the complaint becomes air pollution, a virus, or radiation in a desperate search for any reason to be the cause. But lung cancer is not just a twenty-first century disease—a result of industrial air pollution or smoking—because it also occurred in ancient times when no one smoked, there were no factories or automobiles, and the air was clean.

So, what causes lung cancer? It is a confounding question. Researchers know many people who are diagnosed with lung cancer who live in favorable environmental conditions, but they also are aware of many who smoke and work under very bad environmental conditions (such as in a coal mine) who do *not* get lung cancer.

Medical researchers have discovered that the primary cause of lung cancer is related to the use of tobacco. Cigarettes, cigars, and pipes are all harmful, as carcinogens in tobacco damage cells in the lungs, thus giving smokers a higher risk of lung cancer than nonsmokers.

Another cause of cancer is radon, which comes from soil and rock. Radon is an invisible, odorless, and tasteless radioactive gas. Coal miners can be exposed to radon and, in some areas, radon is even found in homes. Radon detector kits can be used to monitor the radon level in a home.

Asbestos is a group of minerals that occurs naturally, but its fibers can cause cancer. Asbestos fibers are used in certain industries such as construction and they can float in the air, stick to clothes, and break easily into small particles. A single particle of asbestos can affect lung function and will increase the risk of lung cancer.

Exposure to certain air pollutants, like by-products of the combustion of diesel and other fossil fuels, may be related to lung cancer also, however, this relationship has not been clearly defined and requires more research. Other causes are lung diseases such as tuberculosis. Medical studies suggest that scarring incurred from tuberculosis may increase a person's chance of developing lung cancer.

A good environment does not guarantee the prevention of lung cancer, it just decreases the risk.

On the other hand, a bad environmental condition may cause lung cancer and is associated with higher risk, but obviously it is not the *only* factor. I feel that medical research focuses too much of its attention on the environment (an external factor).

Other major factors include internal ones related to the body's immune system and lung function. In my healing theory, the cause of lung cancer is from bioelectricity and the body's biochemicals. External and internal factors, or both, can cause lung cancer.

Treating Lung Cancer

The major treatment for lung cancer is the "Big Three": surgery, radiation, and chemotherapy. Many different treatments and combinations of treatments are used to treat lung cancer—which is chosen depends on the type of cancer, its stage, and the general health of the patient.

Many cancer patients might state that they have never smoked, their surroundings do not have any air pollution, radon, or asbestos, and their families do not have any history of lung disease such as tuberculosis. So why and how do these people develop lung cancer? This is very confusing for experts and patients alike.

In my practice, I have found one thing in common with all lung-cancer patients: a blockage point in the T3 and T6 areas. In my healing system and in

TCM, T3 is the lung-energy point, which is called Lung Shu. If this point has a blockage, the autonomic nerve cannot pass the impulse signal to the lung, and this can cause the lungs to malfunction. If the diaphragm (whose point is T6) is out of balance, it will affect the lungs—this is the internal factor that can cause lung cancer.

But if medical researchers do not consider internal factors, they may never find the real causes of cancer. To research lung cancer with T3 and T6 is simple and does not require huge funding, but to accept a new concept is very difficult for the Western medical community. Western medicine uses a bronchoscopy to locate tumors or blockages—we use a thumb to detect blockages in T3 and T6. Both systems look for blockages related to the disease and it would be beneficial if we could combine our knowledge.

In my healing system, for any lung problem I consider blockages of the diaphragm and the T6. Though the diaphragm has a small range of movement, it will affect the movement of both sides of the lungs.

I believe the diaphragm may be involved in the cause of lung cancer, but, so far in Western medicine, no one has researched the relationship between the diaphragm and lung cancer.

Healing Cancer with the Nervous System

The phrenic nerve, which originates from C3 to C5, controls the diaphragm's function. In medical healing history, this nerve system is only referred to in cases of hiccups. In my healing system, the phrenic nerve relates to any cancerous problem, so it is imperative to open any blockage in this nerve in order to heal any type of cancer. Phrenic nerve blockage is indicated mostly on the LI17 area, and the blockage is usually located on the left side of the neck (even if the lung cancer is located on the right side).

When we release the blockage on LI17, a lung cancer patient may feel the oxygen deep in the lung, chest or abdomen, which TCM calls Dantien, and many syndromes from the lung cancer may be released.

When we use the Tong Ren treatment, we should follow CAT scan reports or X-rays from a doctor's exam to monitor tumor status. If the Tong Ren treatment helps the tumor become smaller or disappear, the patient may be able to avoid surgery. If the tumor stays the same size, the patient can consider waiting on surgery. But if the tumor continues to grow, it is not too late for surgery.

This plan of monitoring tumor size is a sensible treatment plan, but is very difficult to follow because a patient's natural fear of cancer causes them to opt for surgery to remove the tumor as soon as possible. It would be most beneficial if they waited to see the efficacy of the Tong Ren treatment, because they may be able to avoid surgery altogether.

As we know, in Western medical practice, the most common treatment for lung cancer is surgical removal of the tumor and when the tumor is large, surgery is a good option. But some tumors cannot be removed by surgery because of their size or location, and not every patient can undergo surgery because of other medical conditions.

After lung surgery, air and fluids tend to collect in the chest. Common side effects of lung cancer surgery include pain, weakness in the chest and arm, and shortness of breath. Patients may need several weeks, or even months, to regain their energy and strength. If we use Tong Ren treatment (directing the laser beam to the Upper Warmer point CV17 on the acupuncture model), these symptoms can be reduced, and the patient can quickly recover his or her strength from the Chi charge.

Chemotherapy

Another popular treatment for lung cancer is chemotherapy. This technique uses anti-cancer drugs to kill cancer cells in the body. Most anti-cancer drugs are injected into a vein (IV), though some are in pill form. Chemotherapy can be administered intravenously through a catheter, a thin tube which is placed into a large vein and remains there as long as needed.

According to Western medicine, after the cancerous tumor has been removed, cancer cells may still be present in the tissue around the location of the tumor, or elsewhere in the body. Although chemo may be used to control cancer growth or relieve symptoms such as pain, we know that it is a poison, a toxin, and it harmful side effects.

The common side effects of chemotherapy include nausea and vomiting, hair loss, mouth sores, and fatigue. Tong Ren treatment can stop or reduce the side effects of chemotherapy. We just use the laser beam on the Middle and Lower Dantian points: CV12, CV6, and CV4.

Radiation

Radiation therapy is another popular treatment option, sometimes called radiotherapy. It is a technique involving the use of high-energy rays to kill cancer cells. Radiation therapy is directed to a limited area and affects the cancer cells only in that area. Its side effects are not as strong as those from chemotherapy.

There are two ways of using radiation: radiation from a machine is called *external radiation* while radiation coming from an implant placed directly into or near the tumor is called *internal radiation* (the implant is a small container of radioactive material).

As a primary treatment, some doctors use radiation therapy combined with chemo instead of surgery. Radiation therapy may also be used to shrink a tumor before surgery or to destroy cancer cells that remain in the treated area after surgery. An additional use of radiation therapy is to relieve symptoms such as shortness of breath.

Radiation therapy, like chemo, has harmful side effects. Common side effects include: fatigue from the destruction of normal cells (which in TCM indicates the destruction of the Yang Chi); a dry and sore throat (which indicates the destruction of the Yin Chi); difficulty swallowing; skin burning at the site of treatment; and loss of appetite. Most side effects from radiation disappear in time.

With Tong Ren treatment, recovery is quicker. Generally, for healing the side effects of radiation, use the Ouch point on the Tong Ren doll. After the first treatment of about five to ten minutes, the patient should feel a big release, such as breathing easier with the lungs feeling more open, the reduction or cessation of nausea, the cooling of burning skin, and a reduction or complete elimination of pain.

Most patients trust the use of radiation more than the laser beam on the acupuncture model. In fact, these two modalities are doing different jobs, but the laser beam technique is completely free of side effects and can even heal side effects. Radiation guarantees side effects yet does not guarantee killing the cancer cells completely. After radiation treatment in many patients, cancer cells can reappear or they may never have been eradicated in the first place.

Lung cancer often spreads to the brain or bones and doctors may use radiation therapy in the brain or bone on an Ouch point. With Tong Ren we use the laser beam on the Ouch point much like a doctor does, but we use the laser beam on the acupuncture model. For bone treatments, we can tap C6, C7, T1, and the Ouch point with the hammer on the acupuncture model, as well as use the laser beam with any type of lung cancer at any stage. Using the Tong Ren treatment, the non-small-cell and small-cell lung cancers are treated in the same way, because the Chi does its job naturally in both cases.

I often use Tong Ren with a laser beam for any type of cancer and have produced satisfactory results. Western medicine uses a laser for lung-cancer treatment, too, but there is a big difference in our methods and philosophies. Naturally, patients will trust a laser used by doctors in a hospital more than mine.

The use of laser beams in the hospital is a new development in lung cancer treatment called photodynamic therapy. Photodynamic therapy is used for lung cancers that are localized, and it is being studied for use in controlling symptoms in advanced cases when tumors are pressing against other organs, or when patients are too sick to receive other therapies. It uses a special chemical which is injected into the bloodstream where it is absorbed into cells. But whereas the chemical rapidly leaves normal cells, it remains in cancer cells for a longer period of time.

Next, a laser light is pointed at the cancer to activate the chemical and kill the cancer cells that have absorbed it. It is a good idea and works in some lung cancer cases, but it is another way of using chemotherapy's "cell-killing philosophy."

Doctors' treatment of small-cell lung cancer is different than that of other types of lung cancer. In many cases, the cancer cells have already spread to other parts of the body before the disease is diagnosed because small-cell lung cancer spreads more quickly than others do. In order to reach cancer cells throughout the body for healing, chemotherapy is always used. Radiation therapy may also be used, but surgery is part of the treatment plan for only a small number of patients with small-cell lung cancer.

In some cases, patients undergo radiation therapies to prevent tumors from forming in the brain *even though no cancer has been found there*. This treatment is called PCI (prophylactic cranial irradiation), which actually means it is a "just in case" treatment for the prevention of brain tumors.

The use of PCI does not mean that a cancer will not spread to the brain; it may only reduce the risk. But, even before the tumor has spread, the radiation destroys some of the brain's cells, so what is the benefit of using PCI? The use of radiation anywhere within the body will cause a lot of damage and also lower the Chi available for healing.

With Tong Ren therapy, we can use C1, C2, or Yintang points for the prevention of brain tumors. According to my theory, to prevent brain tumors one needs to increase blood circulation in the brain. In Tong Ren healing, small-cell lung cancer responds with a higher healing rate than the non-small-cell variety, but, so far, we have found no explanation for this phenomenon from our practice.

After treatments from a doctor, Tong Ren therapy, or other methods, patients should incorporate preventative techniques in their lifestyle. Of course, to stop smoking is the first piece of advice they will get from any expert. In addition, Tui Na massage can be used on the whole spinal column either weekly or monthly to prevent or heal lung cancer.

With Tui Na, we can focus on C1 and C2 in order to prevent brain problems, and T1 to T7 can activate the immune system and balance biochemicals within the body. Other important Tui Na points are the LI17 and LI18, which keep the vagus nerve and phrenic nerve free. Simple Chi Gong exercises and diet can be important aids as well.

Leukemia

Leukemia is a malignant cancer involving the bone marrow and blood, and described as an uncontrolled growth of blood cells. It can afflict anyone, and it strikes all ages of both sexes. As with all other types of cancer, Western medicine does not know the cause of leukemia. Although chronic exposure to benzene in the workplace and exposure to extraordinary doses of radiation can be causes of the disease, neither of these reasons can explain the majority of cases.

According to a report from the Leukemia Society of America, there were approximately 140,000 leukemia patients in the U.S in 1998. An estimated 245,225 people in the United States are currently living with, or are in remission from, leukemia. In the year 2009, an estimated 44,790 new cases of leukemia were diagnosed in the United States.

Types of Leukemia

The most common types of leukemia in adults are acute myelogenous leukemia (AML), with an estimated 12,810 new cases in 2009, and chronic lymphocytic leukemia (CLL), with about 15,490 new cases reported in that year. Another type—chronic myelogenous leukemia (CML)—is estimated to have affected about 5,050 people in 2009, and the most common type of leukemia in children—acute lymphocytic leukemia (ALL)—was estimated to account for about 5,760 new cases.

Both myelogenous and lymphocytic leukemias can be either acute or chronic. The terms myelogenous or lymphocytic represent the type of cell involved.

No matter what the type of leukemia, the treatment will be the same with the Tong Ren, Tui Na, and Chi Gong treatments.

Symptoms of Leukemia

Acute leukemia progresses rapidly and results in the accumulation of immature, non-functioning cells in the marrow and blood. Because the marrow does not produce enough normal red and white blood cells and platelets, three conditions develop: a deficiency of red blood cells causes all leukemia patients to become anemic; a lack of normal white blood cells hampers the body's immune system; and a shortage of platelets causes bruising and bleeding.

Chronic leukemia progresses at a slower rate since it allows the production of a larger number of mature, functioning cells.

Early signs of chronic lymphocytic leukemia may be fatigue, weight loss, loss of appetite, labored breathing, low-grade fever, a feeling of fullness in the abdomen due to an enlarged spleen, and night sweats. Bacterial infections such as skin infections, fluid accumulation or inflammation of the lungs and sinuses often occur. As the disorder advances, the patient loses the ability to fight off infections.

In later stages of the disease, the liver, spleen, and lymph nodes may steadily increase in size. Chronic lymphocytic leukemia may also invade other tissues such as the skin, the eye socket mucous membrane (which lines the inside of the eyelids), the lungs, the sacs that line the chest, the heart, and the gastrointestinal tract. Swelling and a yellow pigmentation of the skin may also occur.

Cause of Leukemia

No one knows the cause of leukemia, but in my healing system I find one thing in common with all types of leukemia patients, no matter their age or gender: each has a blockage on T7 and T8 on the right-hand side, as well as a major blockage on T1 on one or both sides. I recently discovered that LI17, which is located on the neck, may also have a blockage. When blood cells mutate, they lack oxygen for energy. A low level of oxygen in the body may cause these blood cells to remain in an immature condition. I have treated babies and children who had leukemia and found that they have the same blockages as adults.

Why does a baby get leukemia? Western medical logic and philosophy cannot provide an explanation. Can external factors such as chemicals, radiation, and viruses cause a blockage in the middle of the spinal column in babies, or cause a blockage around the T1, T7, or Ll17 areas? I believe, rather, that a newborn baby may develop a blockage from an injury during delivery, or from an unfavorable position in utero affecting the baby's posture.

Treating Leukemia

Leukemia is one of the easier cancers to treat w th Tui Na, Tong Ren, or Chi Gong therapy. My practice has treated a large number of leukemia patients and experienced a high success rate with them–more than 90% feel much better after their very first treatment. I cannot fully explain why energy-healing is easy and effective treatment for leukemia. It may be because leukemia affects the cells only (no tumor is involved), so the energy does not need to change tumor cells, but change only blood-cell production back to a normal state.

Common sense tells us that any type of cell production requires time, proper bioelectrical energy, oxygen, growth hormone, and nutrition—if any of these factors is missing, the cells will be immature—which is precisely the case in leukemia.

We know that bone marrow problems cause T-cell or white-cell problems. The West's medical protocol for treating leukemia is a bone marrow transplant, yet, this healing method has a high risk and a low success rate. If we can correct the *function* problem of the bone marrow and let the body produce its own normal white cells, then the leukemia should be healed.

So, how can we return bone marrow back to its normal function? In the Tom Tam Healing System, T1 is related to many blood diseases and to bone marrow, which is responsible for producing blood cells. The blockage for bone marrow is around T1 and leukemia patients usually have a puffy area or a mark of some sort on the skin around that area. If we can open this blockage, the leukemia will have a high rate of healing.

Tong Ren is effective in treating leukemia. Before the treatment we should observe the patient's complexion—most are pale. We then apply the TCM's Triple Warmer theory for the Tong Ren treatment using the laser beam on the doll at the Middle Warmer point CV12 or ST21 on the right side. After two to three minutes, the patient's face should turn red, indicating a flow of Chi and better blood circulation.

During treatment, the patient should have an overall feeling of relaxation and warmth. This means the blood and Chi are moving within the body. After ten minutes of a laser beam directed to the Middle Warmer, if the patient is weak, we can turn the laser to the Lower Warmer CV6 or CV4 to charge the Lower Dantian with energy. Sometimes we can use the hammer to stimulate BL9 and T1 on the doll. This technique can open the medullar and cerebella area, which is the connector or passageway for bioelectricity to pass from the brain to the body.

Using Acupuncture

Treatment with acupuncture includes stimulating several areas: T1 and T2 to correct bone marrow function; T7 and T8 on the right-hand side for the promotion of blood circulation; SP6, SP10, and LI11 to support whole-body circulation; and LI17 for balancing the intake oxygen level. Sometimes we need to check C1 on the left side. This treatment has good results, but we still need a doctor's examination to monitor the progress of healing.

Be careful with treating leukemia with acupuncture. Leukemia patients or their families often do not trust acupuncture needles, fearing that they can cause infection. Acupuncture needles are as safe to use as a doctor's knife or a hypodermic syringe, however, psychologically, some patients do not have faith in what we do. We should respect the patient, and if they fear the possibility of infection from needles, we should use either Tong Ren therapy or Chi Gong healing without any physical touch.

Disc Technique

The disc-healing technique requires three or more therapists with the patient sitting in a chair or laying down in a comfortable position. The first step is to put the disc on top of the head covering GV22 and BL6 to activate the growth hormone area. During the discing session, the patient may feel warmth on the head and then a wave of warmth flowing down to the arms or chest as the energy goes down the body.

After a few minutes' charge to open the energy flow on the head, we put the disc on the T1 vertebra, which is the bone-marrow point that opens the energy blockage. At T1 the patient may feel the Chi flow down the spinal column.

The last step is to charge and open the blockage at T7 and T8. Most blockages are on the right-hand side. If a patient uses chemo or other drugs from their doctor, we can use the discing on the kidney area, L2, to clean out the resulting toxins. The whole treatment with discing should take 10 to 15 minutes.

The Role of Diet and Exercise

Diet is an important factor in healing leukemia, and is especially important for patients who consume diet sodas, because they only aggravate the situation. I highly recommend that patients increase the amount of red meat (or any meat) they consume, since the patient needs to replenish the blood cells lost from either the leukemia or one of its conventional treatments.

Many patients supplement their diets with vitamins and minerals. It is better to correct deficiencies in the diet with whole foods, but many people trust pills more than food. Supplements are fine, if an actual vitamin or mineral deficiency has been confirmed by a physician, but should not be depended on otherwise.

Exercise is also important in healing leukemia. Many leukemia patients are too weak to move, but they can meditate or practice a simple, easy Chi Gong form. If possible, a stretch movement around the T1 and T7 areas can help open blockages. For a child, a parent can massage the LI17, T1, and T7 for five to ten minutes a day for healing.

After a Tong Ren, Tui Na, or acupuncture treatment, a medical examination may confirm that the patient is free of leukemia. However, most physicians will still recommend a bone-marrow transplant and/or chemotherapy "just in case."

This reason for treatment is risky, but the family's trust in the doctor combined with the fear of the disease often heavily influence their decision for additional medical treatments. Can children and babies refuse? By law, in America, they must follow the doctor's treatment plan if they are under 18 years old.

When we treat any cancer, including leukemia, we need to combine our techniques with those of modern medicine, because in many cases both are needed: if the patient has anemia, they may need a blood transfusion; if they need nutritional or IV treatment, they must follow their nutritionist's or doctor's advice.

Tong Ren for Cancer Simple Point Chart

Diagnosis	Main Point
	Support Point
Chemo Side Effect	GV20, TW16, LI17, ST12, ST36
	CV13, CV6, BL9, Ouch Point
Radiation Side Effect	BL9, CV6, ST36
	Ouch Point, CV17
Surgery Side Effect	Ouch Point
	CV6, ST36, SP6
Brain	C1, C2, LI17, SI16, Tiandong
	GV20, TW16, LV3, Ouch Point
Brain Stem	GV17, BL9, Tiandong, LI17
	Yiming, ST12, GB20, GV16
Pituitary	GV17, GV22, BL6, Tiandong
	ST12, TW16, TW17
Nasopharyngeal Carcinoma	C3, C4, SI16, SI17, LI17, LI18
	Yintang, LI4, ST12
Larynx	C5, ST10, LI17, Ouch Point
	C4, C6, P7, LI18

Tongue	C5, C6, LI17, LI18
	ST11, LI4
Thyroid Gland	C6, C7, LI18, GV22, BL6
	Ouch Point, K3, LI11, LI4
Parathyroid Gland	C6, C7, LI18, SI16
	Ouch Point, P7, H7
Bone	C6, C7, T1, GV22, Ouch Point
	Hammer from Motor Cortex to S5
Sarcoma	LI17, ST11, T4, T7, K24
	Ouch Point
Thymus Gland	T2, K26, SI16, LI17
	P6, ST12, CV17
Skin	T4, T7, LI17, Ouch Point
	SP6, SP10, LI11
Lung	LI17, ST11, T3, CV17, BL9
	T6, CV4, ST12, LU9
Malignant Lymphoma	T1, T2, T3, ST11, Ouch Point
	T7, SP6, LI18
Multiple Myeloma	C7, T1, T4, T7, LI17

Multiple Myeloma (cont'd)	GV22, Ouch Point
Breast	T2, T4, ST12, LI17, Ouch Point
	GV22, BL6, Ouch Point
Melanoma	T1, T4, T7 Rt
	SP6, BL9, Ouch Point
Heart	T5Lt, LI17, BL9, GV17, ST12
	CV17, P6
Leukemia	T1, T7Rt, T8Rt, ST21, LI17
	T2, SP6, SP10, LI11
Esophagus	T7L, T8Lt, ST12, LI18, Ouch Point
	LI17, ST36, CV13, CV17, P6
Bile duct	LI17, LI18, T9, T10, ST21
	ST12, Ouch Point, ST36, GB34
Stomach	LI18, LI17, T9Lt, CV12
	T8Lt, ST11, ST21, ST36, LV3
Pancreas	LI17, LI18, T7Rt, T8Rt, ST21Rt
	ST10, ST36, GV22, SP6
Colon	T11Lt, T12, LI17, ST12, ST25
	LI18, L4, ST11, CV4, ST37

Rectum	LI17, LI18, T7, L4, L5, S4, S5
	ST12, ST37, T1
Appendix	T11Lt, T12Lt, ST25, LI17, LI18
	ST12, ST37, Ouch Point
Liver	LI17, LI18, T9Rt, ST21Rt, SI17
	ST12, ST11, LV3, GB34
Adrenal	T7, L1, ST12, GV22, LI18
	L2, SP6, BL6, Ouch Point
Kidney	T7, L2, ST11, LI17, LI18
	L1, SP6, LV3, Ouch Point
Cervix	T7, L2, L3, GV22, Ouch Point
	LI17, SP6, CV4, LV3
Ovary	GV22, T7, L3, CV6
	SP6, BL9, LI17, TW16
Vagina	GV22, BL6, LI17, L1, L2, S1, S2
	CV4, SP6, SP9, LV3
Testis	GV22, LI17, L1, T7, Ouch Point
	C1, CV4, SP6, SP9, LV3
Prostate	T7, L3, GV22, CV4, LI17

Prostate (cont'd)	SP6, SP9, S1, S2
Bladder	LI17, LI18, S1, S2, CV4, ST11
	L2, SP9, Ouch Point

Key

C-Cervical	T-Thoracic	L-Lumbar
S-Sacrum	Lt-Left Side	Rt-Right Side
GB-Gall Bladder	ST-Stomach	BL-Bladder
SI-Small Intestine	LI-Large Intestine	SP-Spleen
K-Kidney	LV-Liver	TW-Triple Warmer
H-Heart	P-Pericardium	LU-Lung
CV-Conception Vessel	GV-Governor Vessel	

Using this Theory for Healing Cancer

In order to heal cancer, you must follow the theory. Many people get confused about exactly which acupuncture points they should use, so to make it easy to practice, I have included the common cancer points on this chart.

The first, and very important, piece of information we need is the patient's diagnosis from their medical checkup. If we do not know the diagnosis, we will not know what needs to be healed. This cancer diagnosis must come from a medical doctor who uses standardized tests, including a CT or PET scan, X-ray, an MRI, or, most importantly, a biopsy.

Also, consider this: a written report on the condition of the cancer, based on these tests, sometimes varies, so the final determination should be made by the medical doctor's report, and no other way.

Late-stage cancer may have both primary and secondary tumors involved, formed from main and secondary blockages. We treat the primary first, and consider the secondary after the primary tumor has been resolved.

Both Main and Support points are listed in this chart. Most often, the Main point is an "Ouch" point, an area we can check by hand that is painful to the touch or an area of complaint—this includes the cancer and tumor locations. We need to pay close attention to the Main Ouch points for stimulation.

Sometimes we may see a Cancer of Unknown Primary Origin (CUP). Approximately two to four percent of all cancer patients have a cancer whose primary site has never been identified. In this case, we can focus the treatment on the Ouch point and LI17. Also, we can treat specific symptoms as well, because they may be related to the cancer.

There are many different types of cancer, but for us, the healing theory is the same for all of them. In this chart I did not include rare cancers, because I have not treated them personally; this includes primary bone cancer and primary diaphragm cancer.

However, we can still treat these cancers using this philosophy—we simply need to know which organ contains the cancer and find the blockage in the spinal column related to that organ.

One organ may have more than one type of cancer, yet in the Tom Tam Healing System, this is not important. In general, with our treatment, the main question is: which organ has the cancer? For that affected organ, the treatment will be the same, regardless.

In addition, sometimes we need to consider other factors that may relate to the cancer. Breast cancers like IBC (Inflammatory Breast Cancer) and other types are treated differently. It is necessary to heal the inflammation that relates both to the immune system and to the breast cancer. The liver cancer, if related to Hepatitis C, needs an immune system treatment; if the cancer is related to liver cirrhosis, stimulation of the metabolism system is also needed.

When we treat cancer, understanding the theory is more important than which technique you choose. Each technique's purpose is to open a blockage, and the most important thing is that you choose the technique you're most comfortable using. In the Tom Tam Healing System, we mainly focus on acupuncture, Tui Na, Tong Ren therapy, and Chi Gong healing.

Sometimes a single technique is not enough to open a blockage, so it should be combined with others. For example, if acupuncture cannot reach deep enough to open some blockages, then Tui Na is needed to physically release the tissues. The order in which blockage points are stimulated is not crucial, yet many people focus on the order.

Generally, when we stimulate a nerve, it is from the top down to the bottom; when we stimulate an artery, it begins in the heart and either goes up to the head or down to the leg, depending on where you want to lead the flow of Chi.

In this chart, there are Main points and Support points. We cannot put the details of the Ouch point in the healing chart, because a patient may have more than one Ouch point and the Ouch point can be anywhere on the body. In Tong Ren healing, we simply put the laser on the Ouch point for stimulation.

In my experience in healing cancer, I have found that most patients have a blockage on the left side at LI17—I believe that this phrenic nerve point is the most important point to stimulate. The best technique to open this blockage is Tui Na or another physical healing method—even the patient can use a massage machine or TENS machine to stimulate these points themselves.

The cancer diagnosis and stage, evaluation of the tumor size, and blood markers are all the responsibility of the physician, so the points in this chart are used for healing only, never for diagnosis. For example, when a patient has a blockage in the T4 area, we should not assume that the patient has breast cancer, but every breast cancer patient will have a blockage at T4, because T4 is the pathway of bioelectricity to the breast area.

It is important to remember to include the bladder meridian points to treat the central nervous system. It is not included in the simple cancer point chart because it is not a primary blockage, although it *is* highly beneficial in regulating the brain to generate a relaxation response and to slow down brainwaves. The bladder points from BL1 to BL10 in the skull are necessary in decreasing tight, tender points in soft tissue and in altering brainwaves.

Poll of Tong Ren Healing for Cancer

A pilot study was conducted from September 21 to October 21, 2009. Most of the information was collected from the Haverhill, Burlington, and Quincy, MA, Tong Ren Guinea Pig class locations. All cancer patients who had previously attended one or more Guinea Pig classes were asked to voluntarily complete a survey. Some of the answers were unclear or had missing information. We have many healing classes, and in the future we would like to conduct a larger study, involving more locations and classes.

The purpose of this survey study is to provide some preliminary results to compare with those of various hospital cancer support groups and other cancer healing groups. This study will be a foundation for future studies of cancer and Tong Ren Therapy.

We also did a short-term survey of cancer patients between August 19 and September 5, 2009. This second survey will provide more long-term results. For this study, patients were asked to answer survey questions, then, in three to six months, they were asked again to fill out the same form in order for us to compare the responses.

In this study, we collected 102 forms, over half (53%) of which were indicated as having late-stage cancers diagnosed as either stage 3 or 4 by medical doctors. Only 12% of the study responses were stated as having early stages of cancer, and 35% did not indicate which stage of cancer they had, but we believe that many of these were late-stage. Our experience has shown that early-stage cancer patients rarely join the Tong Ren class.

Massachusetts is renowned as the epicenter of the medical world, with Massachusetts General Hospital and The Dana-Farber Cancer Institute being two major hospitals there noted for healing cancer. In the survey, we asked where patients were being treated and found we have an equal number of patients from these two hospitals.

Many of the oncologists who work in these hospitals know their patients come to see us, yet, according to these patient surveys, only one-third of them support their patients' use of Tong Ren for healing, 45% are ambivalent, and 21% are doubtful of Tong Ren healing.

Poll of Tong Ren Healing for Cancer

(From Sep. 21, 09 – Oct. 21, 09)

Total Cases	102	
Stage 1-2	12	12%
Stage 3-4	54	53%
No information about Stage	36	35%
Hospitals:	Case	
M.G.H	27	26.73%
Dana-Farber	28	27.72%
Others	46	45.54%
Before TR Healing		
Without big 3 ***	41	40%
Used big 3	61	60%

Same time with TR		
Without big 3	64	63%
Used big 3	38	37%
Big 3 used Condition		
Never used big 3	32	31.37%
Using or used big 3	70	68.63%
Type of Cancer in the Poll	Case	
Breast	19	
Colon & Rectum	12	
Pancreatic	7	
Ovarian & Uterine	7	
Lymphoma	7	
Lung	6	
Prostate	6	
Brain	5	
Thyroid	3	
Leukemia	3	
Multiple Myeloma	3	
Melanoma	3	
Others	21	
What you think about TR		
Useless	1	1%
Doubtful	2	2%
Ambivalent	2	2%

Helpful	95	93%
Don't know	2	2%
Total	102	
Provided Doctor's name	78	76%
Told Dr. about TR		
Yes	60	59%
No	36	35%
No answer	6	6%
What Dr. thinks about TR		
Useless	1	2%
Doubtful	12	21%
Ambivalent	26	45%
Support	19	33%
Total	58	
Test before & after TR		
Yes	79	
No	11	
No information	12	
Report from Dr.'s Test		
Worse	8	9.5 %
Stable	17	20.24%
Improved	59	70.24%
*** 3 people have 2 or 3 answers		
Total answer #	84	(79 people)

TR verified by Dr.'s Report	Total	79 Cases
Effective Rate	76	90.5%
Non-effective Rate	8	9.5%

***   Big 3's are Surgery, Chemo, and Radiation

Before beginning Tong Ren healing, 60% of the patients surveyed had used chemotherapy, surgery, and radiation. Some patients used only one of the "Big 3" for healing while others used two or three of the traditional treatments. However, 40% of the patients did not use any chemotherapy, surgery, or radiation before they came to the Tong Ren class. Once people began using Tong Ren healing, 63% of the patients did not use any of the "Big 3," and 37% continued with their "Big 3" treatments.

Many people believe that results of Tong Ren healing are attributable to the "Big 3," particularly chemotherapy. However, in our study it was noted that 31% of the patients (32 cases) never used any of the "Big 3" treatments at all. According to their medical records, out of the 32 cases who never used any "Big 3" treatments, 17 cases have improved and 7 cases are stable. Only 3 cases got worse, and five do not have medical reports from their doctors for comparison.

So, what type of cancer patient should not use the "Big 3" for healing? Or when should patients stop using the "Big 3?" There are so many questions to answer regarding the use of various types of healing methods. Remember, Tong Ren practitioners never advise a patient whether to use the "Big 3" or not; patients in Tong Ren classes make their own decisions regarding the use of medical treatment in conjunction with Tong Ren healing.

Over 18% of patients in this study have breast cancer (19 of the 102 cases) with the second-most prevalent being colon and rectal cancers (12 of the 102 cases). Of these 12 colorectal cancer cases, one was stage 1, and the others were all stage 3 or 4. The third most common cancers in our study are pancreatic, ovarian, and lymphoma, each of which accounted for seven cases.

In our class, all of the pancreatic cancer cases were late stage, yet interestingly enough, these were among the cases with the best results from Tong Ren healing. In the seven cases of pancreatic cancer, one case did not undergo medical testing with a physician, two were reported as 'stable,' and four showed improvement according to their medical tests. Four of these cases have survived more than three years and none indicated in this survey that they were getting worse. In future studies, we wish to focus on such challenging cases. We also would like to conduct another study focusing on breast, colon, and pancreatic cancers.

In our study, 93% of the people who joined the classes believe that Tong Ren healing was "Helpful" to them. Yet, our very high success rate is attributed, by Skeptics, to the "placebo effect" or "coincidence" and "spontaneous." If that is what they would like to call our results, then if the "placebo effect" can make 93% of patients happy, why not use the treatments? I wonder if patients undergoing the "Big 3" feel that their treatment was helpful to them. We cannot definitively state that these high healing results are attributable to the combination of Tong Ren healing and medical care—this will require further study.

Tong Ren healing is relatively new and this survey is only preliminary. Many medical experts and so-called scientists do not accept such surveys—they are only interested in their own way of studying. To a healer, the patient's smile and personal judgment is more valid than a meter's needle or a blinking laboratory light.

In this survey, we found more patients informing their doctors of their participation in Tong Ren healing. After their doctors see their medical tests which indicate that they have improved or become stable, 33% of survey respondents believe that their doctors support their use of Tong Ren healing; 45%

of the doctors are reported to be ambivalent, and 21% had a doubtful reaction. It is significant that one-third of these doctors supported their cancer patients' use of Tong Ren healing—it appears that Western medicine is beginning to realize and accept the benefits of energy healing.

Tong Ren follows a scientific method and theory for healing; its testing must follow modern medical standards. The condition of the cancer (or other diagnosis) must come from standard medical tests performed by medical doctors, not from energy testing or TCM diagnosis. We required all patients who participated in the survey to indicate their diagnosis from medical tests.

This survey had two parts; one before Tong Ren healing and the other after. Also, we plan to wait three to six months for additional medical reports from participating patients so we can compare the results. These results have three possible answers: Worse, Stable, or Improved. In this survey, three people gave two or three answers because a medical report showed that some of their cancers were getting better while others were getting worse. One patient was misdiagnosed because the cancer was stable, but their pain had increased from other, non-cancer reasons.

To date, we have both before and after test reports for 79 people (however, we have 84 answers from these cases). Twenty-three patients required further testing so medical reports could be compared. From the 84 answers received, eight indicated that their cancer had gotten worse (9.5%), 17 showed stability (20.24%), and 59 cases reported improvement (70.24%). According to Western medicine, the reports of stability are signs of good healing which indicate that the treatment is effective. So we count the Stable and Improved as part of our effective rate, for a total of 90.48% of the 84 answers.

Breakdown of eight "Worse" cases from our survey:

Type of Cancer	Case #	Stage	Big 3 before TR	Big 3 During TR
Breast cancer	2	3 & 4	Yes	1 Yes & 1 No
Liver	1	4	Yes	Yes
Sarcoma	1	4	Yes	Yes
Ovarian	1	4	Yes	No
Rectal	1	3	No	No
Prostate	1	1	No	No
Esophageal	1	4	Yes	Yes

In the case of liver cancer, two patients out of the total number indicated that their condition had worsened. In those cases, even though the tumors had decreased in size, the cancer cells were found to still be active, so the doctor diagnosed the case as 'getting worse'. We deferred to the doctor's diagnosis and placed that case in the "Worse" category.

With prostate cancer, the patients followed Tong Ren healing for 10 years. In the beginning, their PSA improved, then it stabilized after a few years, and now it is increasing. In medical studies, as a patient ages, PSA can naturally also increase, so even if the patient's PSA is in the normal range for their age bracket, we still put this case in the "Worse" category.

In the rectal cancer case, a patient was diagnosed two years ago with stage 3 cancer, but refuses to accept any treatment, based on his doctor's advice. According to the patient's last medical report, all indicators had improved, but the patient was still uncomfortable and felt more pain in the abdomen (for reasons other than cancer). In this case, we put it in both the "Worse" and "Improved" categories.

From this chart we can clearly see that Tong Ren therapy did not have an effective rate of 100% for healing cancer—no treatment can claim a success rate that high.

Tong Ren healing should not be classified as alternative medicine; it is complementary medicine—it needs to be combined with other healing methods. A medical doctor's diagnosis is always required and some patients will need antibiotics or alternative treatments from their doctor. But even if the patient is unable to obtain a proper medical diagnosis, Tong Ren healing can still be used to treat their symptoms.

Most cancer patients in our Tong Ren classes combine several healing methods. They may try any (or several) of these options: changing diet, praying, psychic healing, Chi Gong or other type of exercise, taking herbs or vitamins, receiving acupuncture or Tui Na massage, and/or chemo, radiation, or surgery. In these cases, we cannot determine which method actually healed the cancer, because these methods are not covered in our study. We never deny other healing systems for healing cancer, and we do not try to convince our patients to stop other healing treatments.

Many experts try to credit our patient's good healing results to the traditional treatments they received from their practice. We cannot argue with them, yet we would like them to conduct a similar survey of their patients who have not used Tong Ren to see what their effective rate is.

It is difficult to perform a survey about cancer healing with the use of Tong Ren when expert researchers are not available to oversee the study. If we were studying the use of chemicals or herbs to heal cancer, I believe that many experts would be willing to help.

Healing Cancer with the Nervous System

Tong Ren is a new concept of healing which uses the power of the mind to heal many 'incurable' diseases. Its healing range is very wide, making it difficult for people to believe. Of course, this new concept cannot be accepted easily by most healing experts, including those who practice both traditional and alternative medicine.

Many medical experts attack our theories and offer criticism against Tong Ren healing, yet that would never lead us to stop practicing—in fact, quite the opposite. But why are so many experts attacking Tong Ren? It is easy to understand: Tong Ren healing has its own scientific theory, and because it is 'different,' it is often considered 'strange.'

There are many ways to heal cancer—do a search on the Internet and you'll find millions of results. Each healing system resists and denies the others. Tong Ren healers do not fight or deny other healing systems because we believe in scientific evolution. However, the popularity of Tong Ren shows that acceptance is growing quickly.

This survey reports on cancer cases only from our own practice. Some experts have attempted to uncover mistakes in our study method. We encourage the opinions and criticisms of others, because then we learn from them and can correct our mistakes—this allows us to refine our methods for our next study.

Some of the criticisms have nothing to do with science, but come from financial and medical politicians who deny any method of healing that is different from their norm. We have vast experience with these critics, but our interest lies in healing diseases in a scientific way. There is no special honor in practicing Tong Ren healing, yet when we heal patients, especially the "incurable" ones, we are greatly gratified and encouraged to continue our work.

Scientific studies utilize two methods: objective and subjective. So far, the only way to study Tong Ren is objectively. This means if you want to discover healing for yourself, you must join a class to experience it, and talk to other clients or therapists in the class to hear their results and experiences.

This survey is only based on patients' self-reports and medical reports from doctors. We hope, in the future, that we can do double-blind studies of Tong Ren healing.

If you are satisfied with your healing modality and its result, you don't need to come to us—but please do not criticize us. If your condition is not improving, will you give yourself a chance to try another, harmless option? The Tong Ren class doors are open to anyone interested in our healing methods. If you want to know the real story behind these survey results, come join a class.

We never deny the seemingly coincidental and spontaneous nature of our healing approach which we believe flows from the power of the collective unconscious. If Tong Ren can achieve a 90.5% healing rate, why not try this "coincidental" and "spontaneous" approach? At least the probability of success is much higher than the lottery.

What do you think about the Tong Ren class?

Before Tong Ren Class	After Tong Ren Class
Useless	Useless
Doubtful	Doubtful
Ambivalent	Ambivalent
Helpful	Helpful

Afterword

Our first cancer patient was treated in 1992. Of course during these last 18 years, my techniques and theories have been refined, because each year new knowledge is gained and our level of experience develops.

Ten years ago, I began to write my cancer-healing book, *Tong Ren for Cancer.* The current theories are the same, but now there is more information and experience from which to draw conclusions. My basic theory for healing cancer is a combination of the TCM meridian theory and the Western medical theories regarding the nervous system.

The TCM theory does not recognize the nervous system and the Western theories of the nervous system do not accept meridian theories or acupuncture energy points. In fact, they continue to deny and reject each other. Each practitioner or medical expert is loyal to their own medical system—the one that they learned in school. It's difficult for people to change their minds.

I am fortunate to not have attended a medical school to learn Western or Eastern healing systems, so I do not need to be loyal to any one healing system. My mind is carefree; if a healing method is effective, then I follow and use it.

Throughout the world, most cancer experts seek out the causes of cancer—but, unfortunately, they are mainly interested in external factors of cancer. There is no doubt that external factors *can* cause cancer, but these are not the only factors in play—there are internal factors, also.

According to my theory, the nervous system can cause cancer. Forming a theory does not come from arguing with other practitioners or researchers, but from experiencing results—and in order to do this, one must be willing to try different things.

There are many healing support groups in America focused on any of a number of treatment options. Most have financial, political, or religious support. Tong Ren healing groups are growing in America and around the world without financial or religious support; the source of its growth is from the spirit of its followers. Skeptics may want to stop our groups and our practice, but too many patients and their families have experienced healing and believe in the power of Tong Ren.

There is a medical crisis in this country—medical expenses are skyrocketing even as healing rates remain low. There is only one way to solve this problem: we need a healing system that is inexpensive and effective. The answer is the Tom Tam Healing System.

My hope is that you have found this book informative and encouraging. If you are interested in healing cancer, there is only one way to experience it: come join us. This is what science calls objective observation. Our doors are always open.

About the Author

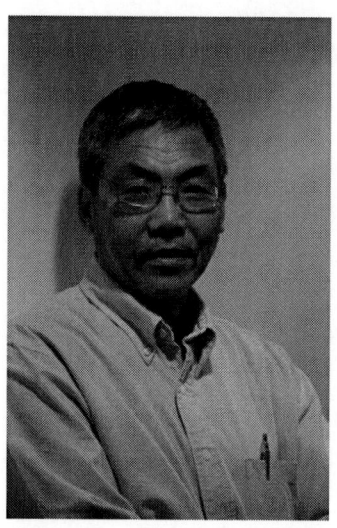

Tom Tam is a writer, poet, and healer. Born in Tai Shan, China, he came to the United States in 1975 as a political refugee. Since 1982, he has been practicing acupuncture, Tai Chi Chuan, and Chi Gong healing with great success. For the last 25 years, Tom has been one of the foremost students of Master Gin Soon Chu, the fifth generation master of the Yang family Tai Chi Chuan.

In 1987, Tom founded the Boston Chi Gong Center and began training students. The following year, he founded the Oriental Culture Institute and organized the Boston Chi Gong Delegation trip to China.

Over the years, Tom has written many books on Chi Gong, healing, and philosophy, including: *Tai Chi Dao Yin* (1993); *Yi Jin Jing* (1994); and *Da Peng Gong* (2000), *Tom Tam Healing System* (1995); *Pi Gu: The Way of Chi Gong Fasting* (1996). In 1994, he developed a new method of healing—Tong Ren Healing—and in 1998 he finished his book, *Tong Ren Therapy: Beyond Acupuncture*. He has written several books of poetry, including *For the Love of Nature* (1997) and *Before the Blooming* (2007). He also authored a translation of *Lao Tzu's Dao De Jing* (1994).

In 1997, Tom completed a book on his approach to past-life therapy, *The Unfinished Life,* and in 1998, he completed two books on his experiences healing patients with cancer: *New Hope on the Horizon* and *Metamorphosis: Emerging from Darkness.*

In 2001 he finished the book, *Tong Ren for Cancer*. In 2002 Tom went to Brazil and observed the Brazilian healer, John of God. He then wrote *Tom Tam in Brazil*. This same year he wrote and published his book about a new concept of psychology: *Chi & Libido*. His most popular book is *A Lazy Bum's Healing* (2003), which has been translated in eight different languages.

In Feb. 2001, he founded the "Guinea Pig" healing class, which is now called the Tong Ren healing class. The Tong Ren healing classes are beginning to get popular in the New England area in America. These Tong Ren healing classes are spreading throughout the world quickly.

Tom Tam is a well known controversial healer worldwide. So far he has received mixed reviews, due to his groundbreaking theories in science and medicine, with more negative criticism than positive awards, depending on one's experience being objective or subjective.

Healing Cancer with the Nervous System (2010) is Tom's latest book, which is the first book in the world that supports the theory that the nervous system can cause cancer. Tom Tam is very satisfied with this book, and is open to comments from readers.

Tom Tam is a carefree dreamer, yet also a tireless, hard worker.